cirencester
college
a beacon college

D0997564

Mastering
the UKCAT

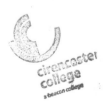

cirencester
college
a beacon college

355274

MASTERING

Mastering the UKCAT: Second Edition
Dr Christopher Nordstrom, George Rendel, Dr Ricardo Tavares
2018

Mastering the BMAT
Dr Christopher Nordstrom, George Rendel, Luke Baxter
2016

Mastering
the UKCAT
Second Edition

Dr Christopher Nordstrom
George Rendel
Dr Ricardo Tavares

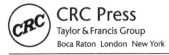

CRC Press
Taylor & Francis Group
Boca Raton London New York

CRC Press is an imprint of the
Taylor & Francis Group, an **informa** business

CRC Press
Taylor & Francis Group
6000 Broken Sound Parkway NW, Suite 300
Boca Raton, FL 33487-2742

© 2018 by Taylor & Francis Group, LLC
CRC Press is an imprint of Taylor & Francis Group, an Informa business.

No claim to original U.S. Government works

Printed by CPI Group (UK) Ltd, Croydon, CR0 4YY on sustainably sourced paper

International Standard Book Number-13: 978-1-1385-9446-3 (Hardback)
International Standard Book Number-13: 978-1-1385-8847-9 (Paperback)

**Visit the Taylor & Francis Web site at
http://www.taylorandfrancis.com**

**and the CRC Press Web site at
http://www.crcpress.com**

Contents

About the Authors

Dr Christopher Nordstrom graduated from University College London with a prize-winning degree in medicine and a first-class honours degree in neuroscience. He undertook medical training in London and now works as a senior doctor in emergency medicine and is a Fellow of the Royal College of Emergency Medicine. Christopher has been involved in medical education for over 10 years, completing a PgCert in Clinical Education and gaining a Fellowship in the Higher Education Academy. He has received written praise for his teaching from hospitals and universities, including Imperial College London and University College London. His academic achievements include publications in world-renowned journals, published original research and regular presentations and national and international conferences. He has also peer-reviewed for the British Medical Journal and is one of the UK's leading UKCAT and BMAT experts, regularly speaking at national events including the Royal Society of Medicine's Career Day.

George Rendel graduated from the University of Leeds with a prize-winning, first-class degree in English. He has used his academic understanding of the English language and his experience in journalism and publishing to become a leading expert in the verbal reasoning and essay writing components of the UKCAT and BMAT examinations. He has worked in educational publishing for Pearson and in consulting for Accenture.

Dr Ricardo Tavares completed his prize-winning Medical Sciences Masters undergraduate degree at Oxford University and went on to finish his medical MBBS training at University College London Medical School. He carried out his foundation training within the Imperial College Deanery before starting specialist registrar training in radiology. Ricardo has several years of experience teaching medicine, both as part of a select group at Imperial College and as a clinical methods teaching tutor for Imperial College medical students. He has been published in leading international journals, spoken at numerous national conferences, and teaches on the clinical MD programme for the University of Buckingham Internal Medicine degree.

Introduction

Background

The United Kingdom Clinical Aptitude Test (UKCAT) was first introduced in 2006. Since its introduction, it has been widely used by medical and dental schools across the UK to aid in the selection of future doctors and dentists. Unlike the traditional A-Level and International Baccalaureate examinations, the UKCAT tests *aptitude*, rather than knowledge. By focusing on innate skills, it is designed to reduce the inequality which may arise between applicants from different backgrounds. This helps to widen access into medicine and dentistry.

The UKCAT consists of a 2-hour computerised test that is administered in test centres across the UK. For international applicants, there are now official test centres in over 135 countries, ensuring almost all candidates have easy access to a testing centre.

You can choose when you sit the examination. Testing dates are available annually from July to the start of October. Each student who takes the examination during this three-month window will get different combinations of questions in each section. This prevents students who sit the examination later from finding out which questions will come up.

> **Top Tip:** We recommend booking your test early, even if you wish to sit it at the end of summer, as test dates fill up quickly and the price increases.

The UKCAT examination consists of five sections, each testing a different skill set. These sections are:

- Verbal Reasoning (VR)
- Decision Making (DM)
- Quantitative Reasoning (QR)
- Abstract Reasoning (AR)
- Situational Judgement Test (SJT)

The Verbal and Quantitative Reasoning sections are logical tests. They assess a candidate's ability to evaluate, problem-solve and draw conclusions, based on written and numerical information.

Abstract Reasoning tests both spatial awareness and pattern recognition. This helps to identify your aptitude for constantly developing and modifying hypotheses. Situational Judgement focuses on presenting students with real-world situations and dilemmas. These are designed to identify how you react and behave in challenging circumstances and cover topics similar to those you will encounter in an interview.

The newest section of the UKCAT, Decision Making, was introduced in 2017. It introduces complex and abstract information and tests your skills of logic and reasoning when making decisions.

Booking Your Test

The UKCAT is not sat in schools or colleges, but at regional Testing Centres. As such, it is best for you to book a test date in a suitable location. Initially, you will need to register online for the test. Registration opens 2 months before the first test date. You can book, reschedule or cancel your appointment through the online system. The price varies depending on the date you choose. In 2018, dates in July and August cost £65; subsequent dates cost £87. The price at international Test Centres outside the UK is higher and the number of available testing dates more restricted.

Bursaries are available for qualifying students, such as those in receipt of the 16–19 Bursary or Educational Maintenance Allowance (EMA), free school meals or from families which meet certain criteria. A full list of criteria and an application form can be found on the UKCAT website.

> **Top Tip:** Book your test date early in the summer, and ensure you have 2 to 4 clear weeks before that date for revision. That way, if you are ill or need to reschedule there is time to spare.

The Test Day

It is essential that you arrive *at least* 15 minutes before the start of your test. This will ensure you register in good time. In addition, if you rush to get there, you will add unnecessary stress to an already tough day.

You need to bring a printout of your confirmation email from Pearson Vue and one piece of photographic identification with you. Once inside, you will be photographed for security reasons and issued with a permanent marker pen and laminated booklet. If you require more space to write you can ask for a supplementary booklet. If you are noise sensitive, they can provide you with ear plugs at the Test Centre.

You are not allowed to bring any personal items into the examination. This includes sweets, drinks and lucky mascots! Everything you need will be provided and you must leave your other belongings in a locker. Once the test has started, you cannot pause or stop the test. If you need a toilet break, this will eat into your test time.

General Exam Format

The test is conducted entirely on the computers provided. The laminated booklets provided are used for calculations and making notes and will be collected at the end, although they will not contribute to your score. The screen is formatted so that the information for each question – text, graphs, tables and so on – is presented on the left hand side of the screen, with the questions themselves on the right hand side.

	Timer Question number
Calculator	Flag for review
Information area	Question area
End exam	Previous Next

Once you have selected an answer, you will click the relevant option, and then the 'next' button to move to the next question. If you are unsure about an answer, you can click on the 'flag' icon to mark it for later. When you reach the end of a section, you have the option to review all questions. There is also a 'review flagged questions' button. This allows you to scroll through only those questions which you have flagged and allows you to use any remaining time efficiently on questions you were unsure about.

You can also navigate through the questions by using keyboard shortcuts. These include:

- *alt + n*: Move to the next question
- *alt + p*: Move to the previous question
- *alt + f*: Flag the current question
- *alt + c*: Open the calculator

Top Tip: Time is your greatest enemy in the UKCAT. Use the 'flag' button sparingly and wisely, to ensure you can quickly scroll through only the questions you were unsure about.

You will have a set amount of time for each question. Once your time is up you will automatically be moved on to the next section. Even if you finish another section early, you cannot go back to an earlier section. The time allocated per section can be seen in the following table:

	UKCAT	UKCATSEN
Verbal Reasoning	22 minutes	27.5 minutes
Decision Making	32 minutes	40 minutes
Quantitative Reasoning	25 minutes	31.25 minutes
Abstract Reasoning	14 minutes	17.5 minutes
Situational Judgement	27 minutes	33.75 minutes
Total	120 minutes	150 minutes

The first minute of each section is reading time. During this time you can read the instructions but not see any questions. For those sitting the UKCATSEN, this is increased to 1.25 minutes.

Most candidates find the time pressure the hardest part of the UKCAT exam. It is therefore essential that when you practice, you do so to time.

UKCATSEN

There is an extended time version of the UKCAT available if you suffer from dyslexia or certain other medical conditions: the United Kingdom Clinical Aptitude Test Special Educational Needs (UKCATSEN). Overall, the UKCATSEN is 25% longer – 150 minutes compared to 120 minutes for the standard test.

You do not need to provide UKCAT with any additional information, as this will be requested by your university directly as part of the application process. You will be required to submit a post-16 year's diagnosis or report recommending additional time in public examinations.

Scoring

The scoring system used in the UKCAT is complicated. The VR, DM, QR and AR sections are each scored between 300 and 900 points. Although each question is worth one mark, the raw scores are scaled to generate a score that is comparable between sections. Situational Judgement is scored differently, with more than one answer potentially scoring marks. For this section, each question is given a 'band' score, ranging from Band 1 (the best) to Band 4 (the worst).

Each section consists of a number of multiple choice questions, with between three and five answer options to choose from. There is no negative marking in any section. So it is essential that you never leave a question unanswered. Even if you do not know the correct answer, you may still guess correctly! In each chapter, we will look at how, if in doubt, you can improve your chances of getting the correct answer by logically eliminating some of the options.

> **Top Tip:** There is no negative marking, so NEVER leave any question unanswered.

You will be presented with a printout of your scores on the day, before leaving the Test Centre. This document will contain your personal details along with your scores for each section. You can also see your total score (between 1,200 and 3,600 points for the four sections scored out of 900 each) and your average score (your total score divided by 4). Once your UCAS application is complete, your chosen universities will automatically be notified of your results. You do not need to send them any additional information.

You can only sit the UKCAT examination once per academic year. Your score is valid for entry to university programmes starting the following academic year (unless you have applied for deferred entry, in which case it is valid for your deferred start date). Unfortunately, if you do not do well at the exam you will need to wait a full year before you can re-sit.

Most universities take the UKCAT into account. But they do so in different ways. This can vary from year to year, so it is essential that you read the latest information on university websites and prospectuses.

Some universities look at certain subsections of the test more closely than others. Some look at the overall score. Some universities have minimum cut-offs, or averages, that you must meet in order to apply. At certain institutions, your UKCAT score will only make up part of your application score; the remaining points will come from your personal statement and A-Level results. Others give out invitations to interview based entirely on UKCAT scores.

The following is a table showing how the scores varied between 2015 and 2017:

	2015	2016	2017
Verbal Reasoning	577	573	570
Decision Making[a]	N/A	N/A	647
Quantitative Reasoning	685	690	695
Abstract Reasoning	640	630	629
Total	**2531**	**1893**	**2540**
Average	**633**	**631**	**635**

[a] Decision Analysis was removed in 2016 and replaced by Decision Making in 2017.

For Situational Judgement in 2017, 28% of candidates scored Band 1, 42% Band 2, 21% Band 3 and 9% Band 4. This ratio has remained almost constant over the last few years.

> **Top Tip:** The last UKCAT testing date is two weeks before the UCAS submission date. Apply to universities where your score will benefit your application the most. For instance, if your score is not as high as you had hoped, then apply to universities which do not focus heavily on UKCAT scores.

General Technique

Although the UKCAT is an aptitude test, it is well-documented that you can significantly boost your score through practice. In this book we will cover specific techniques which you can apply in order to excel in each section. In addition, there are some general techniques which are applicable to all sections.

Every year, general feedback shows that timing is the biggest challenge. The exam is intense. It requires considerable mental stamina to keep the momentum going for the full two hours. It is therefore essential that you 'train' regularly – just like you would for a marathon. In the run up to the exam you should have a structured revision plan, devoting set amounts of time to regular practice. In addition to doing practice questions, you should do timed mock exams which simulate the real exam as much as possible.

When you start doing practice questions it is useful to allow yourself extra time for each question. Once you develop your skills and understand the format you should begin to reduce the time you allocate yourself per question. Eventually, you will complete all questions within the time allowed. By doing questions to time you will ensure that you are as prepared as possible for the test.

As there is no negative marking you must never leave an answer blank. Even if you do not know how to answer a question, there are ways to help improve your odds beyond that of simply guessing. This is a concept that we will develop in later chapters. A blank answer guarantees a score of 0 on that question. An educated guess, on the other hand, provides you with a 1 in 2 to 5 chance of success (depending on the question type).

General Top Tips

- Always practice questions to time.
- Try to simulate the exam conditions when practicing (e.g. do not take breaks, have drinks etc.).
- Understand and use the flag button to ensure you can quickly review questions which you were unsure about.

- Never leave a question blank – there is no negative marking.
- If you are stuck on a question then put down an answer, 'flag' the question and move on.
- Practice allows you to significantly boost your score; set up a structured, intense revision plan 2 to 4 weeks before the exam – and stick to it!
- The exam is tough, so make sure you are well rested the night before and arrive with plenty of time to spare to avoid unnecessary stress.

CHAPTER 1

Verbal Reasoning

Overview

As a doctor, you are committing to a lifetime of learning. This will include regularly reading medical journals, picking out crucial information, and deciding how to modify your practice based on the latest evidence.

There will also be times when you will need to assess critical situations and pick out the key factors in a short span of time. The Verbal Reasoning section of the UKCAT tests your ability to quickly absorb and interpret information.

Format of the Section

This section consists of 11 *Question Sets*. These are each made up of a 200–400 word passage and four associated questions, or 'Items'.

There are two different types of *Question Sets*:

1. *True, False, Can't Tell questions*: Each Item is a short statement. Your task is to say, based purely on the passage provided, whether the statement is 'True' or 'False', or if you 'Can't Tell' whether it is true or false, based on the information given.

2. *Comprehension 'Free Text' questions*: Items can be incomplete statements or short questions. Rather than three set answer options—as with 'True', 'False' or 'Can't Tell'—you are given four 'Free Text' options and must choose one.

You have 22 minutes to complete the Verbal Reasoning section, of which the first minute is reading time. This means that you will have just under 2 minutes per Question Set, or 28.6 seconds per Item.

The time pressure is intense. That is why you need to go into this section with a well-rehearsed strategy.

Logically Follows

Regardless of the Question Set format, it is imperative that your answer reflects only what *logically follows* from the passage.

If something 'logically follows' from the passage, you can't help but reach the conclusion offered, based on the passage alone, without any assumptions or outside knowledge.

For example, let's assume the passage tells us 'in the kitchen there are two apples in the fruit bowl, two in the fridge and no apples anywhere else'. Although not explicitly stated, it would be 'True' to say there are four apples in the kitchen, as this logically follows. However, had the Item said 'there are four apples in the kitchen' and the passage only said 'in the kitchen there are two apples in the fruit bowl and two in the fridge', then the answer would have been 'Can't Tell'. This is because there *might* have been apples somewhere else in the kitchen.

Core Strategy

You can't afford to read the whole passage thoroughly and then address each Item. There simply isn't time! So, when you start a Question Set, leave the passage unread and go straight to the first Item.

The fundamental strategy you should then employ, regardless of the Question Set type, involves six simple steps:

1. Read the statement/incomplete statement/question.
2. Skim the passage for key words and phrases relating to this.
3. Read the sentence(s) containing the key words, as well as those before and after.
4. Continue scanning the passage for further occurrences of the key words.
5. If found again, repeat step 3.
6. Select an answer based on this 'targeted' reading.

These six steps should be repeated for each Item.

That is the bedrock of your approach. Stick to it, and you will put yourself in a strong position to complete the section in time, and start building a respectable score.

To excel, you should tinker your technique according to the *Question Set Format*, develop an understanding of *Clue Words* and what they signify, and recognise the *Common Tricks* that question writers use.

'True'; 'False' or 'Can't Tell'

In order to tackle the 'True'; 'False' or 'Can't Tell' Question Sets effectively, your understanding of each of those three terms must be crystal clear:

True: On the basis of the information in the passage, it logically follows that the statement is true.

False: On the basis of the information in the passage, it logically follows that the statement is false.

Can't Tell: You cannot tell from the information in the passage whether the statement is true or false.

Clue Words

Verbal Reasoning questions are not created by a computer. They are written by human beings. Understanding this point – and taking a few seconds to put yourself in the shoes of the question writer – can often help you reach the correct solution.

In order to make each statement fit neatly into just one of the three options – 'True'; 'False' or 'Can't Tell' – the question writer has to use words that specifically signpost one of those three answers, or that discount the other two.

The vocabulary available to help them do this is quite limited. Therefore, certain words can act as 'clues' as to what the answer might – or might not – be.

There are two types of 'clue' words that are particularly significant:

1. *Definitive words*: Definitive Words are those that help make a statement 'black and white'. They tend to shut down multiple possibilities and leave us with only one viable option. These include: 'impossible'; 'cannot'; 'never'; 'only'; 'solely'; 'certainly'; 'exclusively'; 'must' and 'always'.

   For example, the statement 'Ferraris are only red' leaves no room for doubt as to what colour a Ferrari is.

2. *Mitigating words*: Mitigating Words are those that make a statement less definitive and introduce 'shades of grey'. They tend to open up multiple possibilities. These include: 'might'; 'could'; 'can'; 'sometimes'; 'often'; 'frequently'; 'likely' and 'rarely'.

   For example, the statement 'Ferraris are *sometimes* red' opens up the possibility that Ferraris could be blue, black, silver and so on.

These 'clue' words won't automatically give you to the right answer. But they should act as red flags and prompt you to ask yourself:

'Why has the question writer included these words in the statement, or in the relevant part of the passage?'

They are not there by mistake; they are serving a purpose. Therefore, you should view them as signposts to guide you towards the right answer. Often, it is the presence of these words that will ultimately signal whether the answer is 'True', 'False' or 'Can't Tell'.

On the surface, Mitigating Words lend themselves more to 'Can't Tell', while Definitive Words lean towards 'True' or 'False'.

But more important is whether the *type* of 'clue' words – definitive or mitigating – in the statement match those in the corresponding part of the passage.

Example 1

The statement is definitive, but the relevant part of the passage is mitigated. Or the statement is mitigated, but the relevant part of the passage is definitive. This *mismatch* often means that the likely answer is either 'False' or 'Can't Tell'.

Statement: Ferrari *never* makes blue cars [definitive].

Relevant part of passage: Ferrari *usually* makes red cars [mitigated].

Answer: Can't Tell.

Example 2

If the statement and the relevant part of the passage are *both* either definitive or mitigated, this *match* often lends itself to a 'True' or 'False' answer.

Statement: Ferrari *solely* makes red cars [definitive].

Relevant part of passage: Ferrari *never* makes cars that are not red [definitive].

Answer: True.

Top Tip: Look out for definitive and mitigating 'clue' words. Ask yourself why the question writer included them. Check if the type of 'clue' words in the statement and the passage match.

Common Tricks

In the Verbal Reasoning section, there are a number of 'tricks' that question writers can use to catch you off guard. Over the next few pages, we are going to demonstrate these through example questions.

Each question will use a common 'trick'. Do your best to answer all questions within each set before reading the explanations. Once you are aware of the main 'tricks', and the mechanics of how they work, you will quickly learn how to recognise and overcome them in exam situations.

Refer to the following *Example Set 1*. Using the *six-step strategy* and looking out for *clue words*, answer all four questions in 2 minutes. Make a note of your answers before moving on to the explanations.

Example Set 1

Scientology is a body of beliefs and practices started in 1952 by science fiction writer L. Ron Hubbard. Hubbard was succeeded by the current leader of Scientology, David Miscavige, in 1987.

The Church of Scientology was granted tax exemption by the US Inland Revenue Service in 1993, on this basis that it was a 'religion'. Scientology is also recognised as a religion by countries including Sweden, Spain and Portugal. However, other nations, like Canada and the United Kingdom, do not afford Scientology religious recognition. Many people go as far as to suggest that it is a cult, and, moreover, that it brainwashes and extorts its followers. This might be because it is impossible to ascend the ranks of the Church of Scientology without paying cash to advance through the various levels, which range from 'Clear' to 'Operating Thetan' Levels I through XV.

It can be widely read on the internet (which practising Scientologists are deterred from using), that Scientology scriptures make reference to a character named Xenu. As dictator of the 'Galactic Confederacy', Xenu supposedly brought billions of his people to Earth 75-million years ago, stacked them around volcanoes and killed them using hydrogen bombs. Some ex-Scientologists have said that the Church of Scientology only tells its followers about Xenu when they reach Operating Thetan Level III.

Perhaps the most famous practitioner of Scientology is Tom Cruise, who is an Operating Thetan Level VII. David Miscavige was Tom Cruise's best man at his wedding to Katie Holmes in 2006. Cruise has spoken in favour of the Church of Scientology many times since joining in it in 1990.

1. The leader of Scientology was Tom Cruise's best man in his marriage to Katie Holmes

    A.   True

    B.   False

    C.   Can't Tell

2. Tom Cruise has been told about Xenu by the Church of Scientology

    A.   True

    B.   False

    C.   Can't Tell

3. The Church of Scientology is not exempt from paying taxes in Canada and the UK

    A.   True

    B.   False

    C.   Can't Tell

4. Actor Tom Cruise is arguably the most famous practitioner of Scientology

    A.   True

    B.   False

    C.   Can't Tell

Example Set 1: Answers and Explanations

Question 1

The leader of Scientology was Tom Cruise's best man in his marriage to Katie Holmes

ANSWER: 'True'

We know from the last paragraph that David Miscavige was Tom Cruise's best man at his wedding to Katie Holmes in 2006. We also know from the first paragraph that David Miscavige is the current leader of Scientology, and has been since succeeding L. Ron Hubbard in 1987.

This question is a demonstration of *Dispersion of Key Words*.

Dispersion of Key Words

Question writers know you will be scanning the passage for the key word(s) from the statement. This is a common strategy. When there is only one mention of the key word(s) in the passage, it makes life easier. But question writers don't always want your life to be easy! So they sometimes make things harder ensuring that:

1. The same key word/phrase is used in different places throughout the passage.

2. Different keys words/phrases from the statement are scattered throughout the passage.

In this example, the key word is 'David Miscavige'. Scanning for this word, we see that it is mentioned in the second sentence. However, it is important to *keep scanning* for all mentions of the key word throughout the passage. Otherwise, we might miss crucial information that confirms, mitigates or – as in this case – elaborates on the information we already have.

Example Set 1: Answers and Explanations

Question 2

Tom Cruise has been told about Xenu by the Church of Scientology

ANSWER: 'Can't Tell'

From the third paragraph, we know that 'some ex-Scientologists' have said that the Church of Scientology tells its followers about Xenu at Operating Thetan Level III. Tom Cruise is an Operating Thetan Level VII. So, if the ex-Scientologists referred to are telling the truth, then Tom Cruise would have been told about Xenu by the Church of Scientology.

However, in the phrase '*some* ex-Scientologists', the word 'some' is a clear mitigation. We cannot assume that something is true, just because 'some' people have said it. Furthermore, the fact that we are only told what has been said, rather than what definitively *is*, represents a further form of mitigation, confirming that the correct answer is 'Can't Tell'.

This question is a demonstration of *Mitigation*.

Mitigation and Contradiction

Mitigation and Contradiction occur when one part of the passage appears to confirm the statement as 'True' or 'False', only for another part of the passage to provide further information that challenges this.

Mitigation or contradiction can occur within the same sentence as the key word(s) from the statement. But sometimes, mitigation or contradiction comes in the sentence before or after. So, make sure that you scan the sentences that precede and follow the one containing your key word(s) – just in case! If mitigation or contradiction occurs elsewhere in the passage, hopefully your search for dispersed key word(s) will lead you to it.

Example Set 1: Answers and Explanations

Question 3

The Church of Scientology is not exempt from paying taxes in Canada and the UK

ANSWER: 'Can't Tell'

We know that the Church of Scientology is exempt from paying taxes in the US because the Inland Revenue Service recognises it as a religion. We know that the UK and Canada do not recognise it as a religion. But this does not prohibit it being exempt from paying taxes in those countries for some other reason.

This question is a demonstration of *Faulty Logic*.

Faulty Logic

Faulty logic occurs when the *structure* of the argument employed does not make logical sense. This can lead to reasonable premises – in terms of content – being used to justify an unsound conclusion. There are some common examples of faulty logic that tend to recur in the Verbal Reasoning section of the UKCAT. A key piece of logic to remember is:

If X means Y, then Y does not necessarily mean X.

Example: *All humans are mammals, but not all mammals are human.*

Causation is another logic-related pitfall. So, whenever causation comes up, that should act as a red flag. The question writer will often try to tempt you into *assuming* a causal relationship between two things in the passage, where such a relationship does not logically follow.

Example: *Saying that many people who eat a lot of chocolate suffer frequent headaches is not the same as saying that eating chocolate causes headaches!*

Top Tip: Remember: Just because many people who do X also do/have/are Y, we cannot assume that X causes Y (unless stated explicitly in the passage.)

Example Set 1: Answers and Explanations

Question 4

Actor Tom Cruise is arguably the most famous practitioner of Scientology

ANSWER: Can't Tell

In the final paragraph, we read that: 'perhaps the most famous practitioner of Scientology is Tom Cruise'. This appears to corroborate the statement. However, nowhere in the passage are we told that Tom Cruise is an 'actor'. Nor is the possibility excluded. So we cannot tell from the information given whether or not the statement is 'True' or 'False'.

This question is a demonstration of *Outside Knowledge*.

Outside Knowledge

You should NEVER bring outside knowledge into your reasoning. Remember:

'It is important to base your answer only on the information in the passage and not on any other knowledge you may have'.

Question writers might try to trick you into using outside knowledge. They can do this by throwing in something that you will almost certainly know, but that does not follow logically from the passage. In the previous example, you will know that Tom Cruise is an actor, but it is not stated in the passage and is not a logical inference.

Another way to lure you into using outside knowledge is to appeal to your ego. If you have good general knowledge, it's natural to want to show this off. For instance, if you are told that a vessel was travelling at 770 miles/hour, you might be tempted to say it is 'True' that the vessel in question broke the sound barrier. But unless we are explicitly told in the passage that this happened, or that the speed barrier is 767 miles/hour, the actual answer would be 'Can't Tell'.

Top Tip: If they refer to something you know, but it is not explicitly stated within the passage, don't fall for it!

To demonstrate the next common 'tricks', we're going to use a different passage. Please refer to *Example Set 2*, in the following. As before, use the *six-step strategy* and look out for *clue words*. There are only two questions in this set, so you have just 1 minute to finish both. Make a note of your answers to all questions before moving on to the explanations.

Example Set 2

Lance Armstrong was one of the world's most celebrated sportsmen, having won seven consecutive *Tour de France* races between 1999 and 2005. This feat was all the more remarkable as it came after he was diagnosed with advanced testicular cancer in 1996. Armstrong undeniably achieved things that have never been matched before or since, and was respected as much for his work off the bike as on it. In 1997, he launched the Lance Armstrong Foundation to provide support to Cancer sufferers. The name of the foundation was changed to Livestrong in 2003.

Rumours had long circulated that Armstrong might have been involved with doping. These rumours had always been fiercely rebuffed by Armstrong and his representatives. For example, he successfully sued *The Sunday Times* and its writer David Walsh for alleging that he had cheated during his *Tour* successes. However, in 2012 Armstrong was given a lifetime ban by the United States Anti-Doping Agency (USADA). He was also accused of running 'the most sophisticated, professionalised and successful doping program that sport has ever seen'.

After initial protestations, Armstrong admitted to taking banned substances when he appeared on the *Oprah Winfrey Show* in January 2013. There were a number of legal consequences to this admission. Among others, Armstrong was sued by SCA Promotions for the $12 million it paid out insuring his *Tour* wins, and was also counter-sued by the *Sunday Times*.

1. Armstrong's achievements were unique

   A. True

   B. False

   C. Can't Tell

2. USADA accused Armstrong of running 'the most sophisticated, professionalised and successful doping program that sport has ever seen'

   A. True

   B. False

   C. Can't Tell

Example Set 2: Answers and Explanations

Question 1

Armstrong's achievements were unique

ANSWER: True

The word 'unique' does not arise in the passage. However, we are told that Armstrong 'undeniably achieved things that have never been matched before or since'. The fact that this is 'undeniable' means that it is certain. And saying that his achievements have 'never been matched before or since' is effectively synonymous with saying that they were 'unique'.

This question is a demonstration of *Synonyms*.

Synonyms

We have already examined the way question writers can make the 'skimming' strategy more challenging by *Dispersion of Key Words and Phrases* throughout the passage.

Another – even trickier – technique they can employ to throw you off is to use synonymous words or phrases in the passage, rather than the precise ones from the statement. This means that you can't simply look for the same word; you also need to be aware of words which mean the same thing. Since this requires more interpretation, it becomes a more difficult task.

Usually, you won't have to worry, as there will be some identical vocabulary from the statement to signal the relevant part of the passage. This will give you the foothold you need to ensure you are in the right place. But, just occasionally, that won't be the case. Ultimately, this means that you have to look for both:

1. Key words/phrases

2. Synonymous key words/phrases

Of course, you will not be able to think of *all* synonymous words and phrases and skim the passage looking for them. That wouldn't be very time efficient at all. But what you can do is take a mental note of words or expressions that have a similar meaning. If you don't find the specific word in question, then these similar words/expressions will be your next port of call.

> **Top Tip:** You can also use other key words as a guide. In the earlier example, looking for 'achievements' will take you to 'achieved'. By reading around this, you will notice that the subsequent wording makes clear that the achievements referred to were unique.

Example Set 2: Answers and Explanations

Question 2

USADA accused Armstrong of running 'the most sophisticated, professionalised and successful doping program that sport has ever seen'

ANSWER: Can't Tell

Reference to USADA is made in the second paragraph. We are told that they gave Armstrong a lifelong ban in 2012. The next sentence has the crucial quote about 'running the most sophisticated, professionalised and successful doping program that sport has ever seen'. But, while USADA are mentioned in the preceding sentence, these words are not attributed to USADA. Nor are they attributed to anyone else. Therefore, we Can't Tell if they came from USADA or not.

This question is a demonstration of *Juxtaposition*.

Juxtaposition

Juxtaposition occurs when two ideas or objects are placed next to each other within the passage. The key thing to remember is that just because two things are stated in close proximity, it does not mean that they are linked – even if they refer to similar topics and use similar language.

Question writers will often include two statements side-by-side, hoping that you will *assume* a link between them that is not explicitly stated, and does not logically follow from the passage. In order to avoid this pitfall, there are some simple DOs and DON'Ts that you should adhere to:

> *Do*: Look for *bridging phrases*. These are short phrases that suggest a genuine and explicit link between two pieces of information. They include: 'because of'; 'due to'; and 'as a result of'. When you see these – or similar phrases – they often suggest a link and/or a causal relationship between two things.

> *Do not*: *Assume* that two statements are linked, or have a causal relationship. That they relate to the same theme is not enough. In order to logically infer a link and/or a causal relationship, the passage must make the link explicit – usually by employing a *bridging phrase*.

Recall our example of assumed causation when we discussed *Faulty Logic*:

Saying that many people who eat a lot of chocolate suffer frequent headaches is not the same as saying that eating chocolate causes headaches!

Read the following statement:

'Chocolate causes headaches'.

Now, consider whether that statement is 'True', 'False', or if you 'Can't Tell', based first on Sample 1, and then on Sample 2.

Sample 1

A study was conducted on people who suffer an above-average amount of headaches. These people were given a survey about their life style. The survey showed that they also ate an above-average amount of chocolate.

'Chocolate causes headaches'.

    A. True

    B. False

    C. Can't Tell

Sample 2

A study was conducted on people who suffer an above-average amount of headaches. These people were given a survey about their life style. A scientific experiment proved that the frequency of their headaches was a result of the fact they also ate an above-average amount of chocolate.

'Chocolate causes headaches'.

    A. True

    B. False

    C. Can't Tell

What did you say? The correct answers are:

Sample 1: 'Can't Tell'

Though we are told that the people who suffered an above-average number of headaches also ate an above-average amount of chocolate, there is nothing to logically infer a link between the two. We can't assume that chocolate causes the headaches, because there could be any number of other factors involved. The chocolate could be a mere coincidence. There are no bridging phrases linking the two things, or establishing a causal relationship.

Sample 2: 'True'

In this case, we have a clear bridging phrase – 'was a result of' – that establishes a causal relationship between the chocolate and the headaches. We also have definitive language: this relationship was 'proved'.

> **Top Tip:** Look for *bridging phrases* that signpost a causal relationship. Don't assume links/causal relationships based on juxtaposition!

To demonstrate the next common 'tricks', we're going to use a different passage. Please refer to the following *Example Set 3*. As before, use the *six-step strategy* and look out for *clue words*. There are only two questions in this set, so you have just 1 minute to finish both. Make a note of your answers to all questions before moving on to the explanations.

Example Set 3

Amanda Knox served 4-years in prison in Italy for the murder of Meredith Kercher in Perugia in 2007. The trial was covered extensively by media around the world. There are many reasons for this, including the unusual and macabre nature of the murder of the young English student. But the centre of attention was undeniably Knox herself, whose youth, good looks and often strange behaviour before and during the murder trial, made her both famous and infamous. Also convicted of the murder was Knox's then boyfriend, Raffaele Sollecito, who was given a 25-year sentence – one year less than Knox.

Knox and her legal team had always pointed to a number of inconsistencies in the case against her. The defence repeatedly cited the possible contamination of DNA evidence used against her, as well as her treatment during questioning. This was allegedly aggressive, and conducted over many consecutive hours in Italian: a language that Knox did not then understand fluently. In 2009, her family told the *Sunday Times* that Knox had not been given an interpreter.

Knox and Sollecito's convictions were overturned on 3 October 2011 after a second appeal. The decision was based largely on a 145-page report questioning the validity of the DNA evidence. The hearing was conducted solely in Italian, and Knox spoke in detail, clearly and cohesively, when called upon. After being released, Knox returned to the US, where she lives with her family. However, her acquittal was overturned in March 2013, and the case will go back to court. If she is found guilty, the Italian authorities could demand her extradition from the US.

1. Amanda Knox speaks Italian well

    A.   True

    B.   False

    C.   Can't Tell

2. Amanda Knox was given a sentence of at least 26 years

    A.   True

    B.   False

    C.   Can't Tell

Example Set 3: Answers and Explanations

Question 1

Amanda Knox speaks Italian well

ANSWER: True

In the third paragraph, we are told that: 'The hearing was conducted *solely* in Italian, and that Knox spoke in detail, clearly and cohesively, when called upon'. The key word is 'solely'. If the only language spoken was Italian and Knox was able to speak with detail, clarity and cohesion, it is fair to infer that she speaks Italian well.

There is a red herring in the second paragraph, when reference is made to her being questioned in a language 'Knox did not then understand fluently'. But the key mitigating word is 'then', making the statement historical. It is superseded by the information in the last paragraph.

This question is a demonstration of a statement that *Sounds Like Can't Tell* (but isn't!).

Sounds Like Can't Tell

There are a couple of sneaky ways of making a statement seem like an obvious 'Can't Tell' when, in fact, it is 'True' or 'False'. This includes the absence from the statement, passage, or both, of key words, combined with the use of subjective words that seem like they will be hard to confirm or refute.

We can combat the absence of key words by being particularly vigilant for *Synonyms* – those words and phrases that mean the same as something in the statement, even if the vocabulary is not identical.

Using subjective terms primes us to select a 'Can't Tell' answer. In the earlier example, it is easy to think: 'How do you define speaking Italian "well"?' We might think that this is not possible, and quickly guess at 'Can't Tell'. But, as shown by the explanation, it is possible to make a *value judgement* from logical inference.

Example Set 3: Answers and Explanations

Question 2

Amanda Knox was given a sentence of at least 26 years

ANSWER: False

We know from the end of the first paragraph that Raffaele Sollecito was given a 25-year sentence and that this was 'one less than Knox'. We can therefore calculate, from the information given, that she was given a sentence of *exactly* 26 years. To say the sentence was 'at least 26 years' is therefore false.

This is an example of statements that use *Numbers*.

Numbers

Basic calculations are a form of logical inference. So be prepared to do quick additions, subtractions and multiplications in your head to arrive at the right answer. For example:

'In the kitchen, there are two apples in the fruit bowl and two apples in the fridge, and no apples anywhere else'.

Based on this information, it would be 'True' to say that there are four apples in the kitchen, as this does follow logically from the passage.

'Averages' come up quite frequently in the Verbal Reasoning section. There is a trick associated with averages that can be explained through the following example:

You are told that the average height of boys in a sixth form class is 170 centimetres. You might, therefore, assume that it is 'True' that some boys are shorter and some taller than 170 centimetres. However, it is *possible* (unless specifically discounted) that *all* the boys are exactly 170 centimetres. So the answer to the statement: 'one or more boys are shorter/taller than 170 centimetres' is actually 'Can't Tell'.

> **Top Tip:** When an average is given, remember that as well as numbers below and above, there might be numbers that are *exactly equal* to this average.

Summary of Common Tricks

1. Dispersion of key words
2. Mitigation and contradiction
3. Faulty logic
4. Outside knowledge
5. Juxtaposition
6. Synonyms
7. Sounds like 'Can't Tell'
8. Numbers and averages

Free Text Comprehension Question Sets

'Free Text' Question Sets were introduced in 2013. They now make up a significant percentage of the Verbal Reasoning section. In fact, in recent years, they form the majority of questions, typically 7 out of the 11 question sets.

It is first worth noting what is the same, and what is different, in the 'Free Text' format.

What's the Same?

- The passage – same length and topic types
- Number of items per passage – still four
- Key principals – still what 'logically follows'
- Common tricks – same ones... plus a few more!

What's Different?

True, False, Can't Tell	Free Text
Items are complete statements	Items are incomplete statements/questions
Three answer options	Four answer options
Always 'True', 'False' or 'Can't Tell'	Possible answers are free text
Time pressured	Even more time pressured!

Strategy

You can still follow the core, six-step strategy. However, there are some nuances you can add to improve results for this format:

1. Skim passage for the key words/phrases from the question/incomplete statement.

2. Read around those key words/phrases to gain a high level sense of what the passage has to say on that topic.

3. Read the answer options one-by-one, cross-referencing against the relevant part of the passage where needed.

4. Discount non-viable options straight away

   - If you reach a perfect fit, select it and move on.
   - If there is no perfect fit, assess all options and choose best.

Item Types

Before 2013, when all the Items asked if the statement was 'True', 'False' or 'Can't Tell', you knew exactly what to expect. That's no longer the case. In the 'Free Text' format, each answer option can say pretty much anything. It may seem that the possibilities are endless.

However, in reality, Items within this Question Set format generally fall into one of a limited number of categories. You can be asked to identify:

- The correct ending to incomplete statements
- Whether something is true/false

- Conclusions/definitions from the passage
- Causes/consequences of certain things

And though they might try to muddy the water by asking you to make Value Judgements, your strategy will largely remain the same.

We are now going to tackle each of these Item categories with some more worked-through examples.

Please refer to Example Set 4, in the following. The passage is similar to the one used in *Example Set 3*, but there are key differences, so be careful! There is only one Question in this set, so try to answer it in *30 seconds*.

Example Set 4

Amanda Knox served 4 years in prison in Italy for the murder of Meredith Kercher in Perugia in 2007. The trial was covered extensively by media around the world. There are many reasons for this, including the unusual and macabre nature of the murder of the young English student. But the centre of attention was undeniably Knox herself, whose youth, good looks and often strange behaviour before and during the murder trial, made her both famous and infamous. Also convicted of the murder was Knox's then boyfriend, Raffaele Sollecito, who was given a 25-year sentence – one year less than Knox.

Knox and her legal team had always pointed to a number of inconsistencies in the case against her. The defence repeatedly cited the possible contamination of DNA evidence used against her, as well as her treatment during questioning. This was allegedly aggressive, and conducted over many consecutive hours in Italian: a language that Knox did not then understand fluently. In 2009, her family told the *Sunday Times* that Knox had not been given an interpreter.

Knox and Sollecito's convictions were overturned on 3 October 2011 after a second appeal. The decision was based largely on a 145-page report questioning the validity of the DNA evidence. The hearing was conducted solely in Italian, and Knox spoke in detail, clearly and cohesively, when called upon. After being released, Knox returned to the US, where she lives with her family. However, her acquittal was overturned in March 2013, and the case will go back to court. If she is found guilty, the Italian authorities could demand her extradition from the US.

Knox's conviction was overturned mainly because:

    A. The trial was a centre of media attention around the world.

    B. She was treated aggressively when questioned.

    C. The DNA evidence was false.

    D. A report raised questions about some of the evidence.

Example Set 4: Answers and Explanations

Answer: D

The key part of the passage is: 'Knox and Sollecito's convictions were overturned on 3 October 2011 after a second appeal. The decision was based largely on a 145-page report questioning the validity of the DNA evidence'.

Since the decision to overturn was based 'largely' on this report we know that the report was the main reason. Since it questions the validity of the DNA evidence, it clearly questioned the evidence. And since it was significant enough to get the decision overturned, we can also infer that the evidence was 'key'.

This an example of an *Incomplete Statement*, which is the most common Item type in the free text format.

Incomplete Statement

Often, you will be presented with incomplete sentences and asked to select the right ending. For example:

- 'Mercury has not been extensively studied because'
- 'Poverty is a relative measure because'

When faced with this format, you should treat each answer option as a mini 'True', 'False' or 'Can't Tell' task.

Only if the complete sentence – the partial statement ending with the given answer option – is 'True', is that answer correct.

Please refer to *Example Set 5*, in the following. The passage will be familiar – but the questions won't! There are four questions in this set, so you have 2 minutes to finish. Make a note of your answers to all questions before moving on to the explanations.

Example Set 5

Scientology is a body of beliefs and practices, started in 1952 by science fiction writer L. Ron Hubbard. Hubbard was succeeded by the current leader of Scientology, David Miscavige, in 1987.

The Church of Scientology was granted tax exemption by the US Inland Revenue Service in 1993, on this basis that it was a 'religion'. Scientology is also recognised as a religion by countries including Sweden, Spain and Portugal. However, other nations, like Canada and the United Kingdom, do not afford Scientology religious recognition. Many people go as far as to suggest that it is a cult, and, moreover, that it brainwashes and extorts its followers. This might be because it is impossible to ascend the ranks of the Church of Scientology without paying cash to advance through the various levels, which range from Clear to Operating Thetan Levels I through XV.

It can be widely read on the internet (which practising Scientologists are deterred from using), that Scientology scriptures make reference to a character named Xenu. As dictator of the 'Galactic Confederacy', Xenu supposedly brought billions of his people to Earth 75-million years ago, stacked them around volcanoes and killed them using hydrogen bombs. Some ex-Scientologists have said that the Church of Scientology only tells its followers about Xenu when they reach Operating Thetan Level III.

Perhaps the most famous practitioner of Scientology is Tom Cruise, who is an Operating Thetan Level VII. David Miscavige was Tom Cruise's best man at his wedding to Katie Holmes in 2006. Cruise has spoken in favour of the Church of Scientology many times since joining in it in 1990.

1. If the passage is true, which of the following statements is also true?

    A.   Tom Cruise has paid money to the Church of Scientology.

    B.   L. Ron Hubbard died in 1987.

    C.   There are many Scientologists in Spain.

    D.   Canada and the UK have the same tax system.

2. Based on the passage, which of the following statements is most likely to be true?

    A.   David Miscavige is related to L. Ron Hubbard.

    B.   Reference to Xenu is easily found online.

    C.   Scientologists never go on the internet.

    D.   Katie Holmes is a scientologist.

3. Which of the following statements, if true, would weaken the argument that Scientology is a cult?

    A.   Senior Scientologists claim they have not been brainwashed.

    B.   Senior Scientologists have not paid any money to the Church of Scientology.

C. Scientology is granted tax exemptions in over 20 countries.

D. Scientology does not completely ban followers from using the internet.

4. Which of the following conclusions about Scientology can be drawn from the passage?

A. Scientology is based on the science fiction of L. Ron Hubbard.

B. Scientology is a cult.

C. Scientology is recognised as a religion in some countries but not others.

D. Scientology actively looks to recruit celebrity followers.

Example Set 5: Answers and Explanations

Question 1

ANSWER: A

Looking for key words, we learn that levels of Scientology range from Clear to Operating Thetan Levels I through XV'. We know that Tom Cruise is an Operating Thetan Level VII. We also know that 'it is impossible to ascend the ranks of the Church of Scientology without paying cash to advance through the various levels'. Therefore, in order to have reached Operating Thetan Level VII, Tom Cruise must have given money to the Church of Scientology.

This is an example of a *Free Text True or False*.

Free Text True or False

In the free text question sets, you might still be asked whether something is true or false. When this happens, you can apply the same principles that have been established for the 'True', 'False' or 'Can't Tell' format.

Common examples:

- Which of the following is/is always true?
- If the passage is true, which of the following is also true?
- Which of the following is most/least likely to be true?

In order to find the right answer, you should employ the following strategy:

1. Use exactly the same methodology as the 'True', 'False', 'Can't Tell'.

2. It is only 'True' if it logically follows with no assumptions.

3. Treat each option like a mini 'True', 'False', 'Can't Tell' exercise.

4. Stop when you find a logically perfect answer.

Example Set 5: Answers and Explanations

Question 2

ANSWER: B

1. We only know that David Miscavige succeeded L. Ron Hubbard as leader of Scientology. This does not mean they are related.

2. We are told that it can be 'widely read on the internet' that there is a character called Xenu in the Scientology Scriptures. For this to be the case, it is likely to be true that references to Xenu are common online.

3. Though we know that Scientologists are 'deterred from using' the internet, this does not mean they never do so.

4. We know only that Tom Cruise is a Scientologist and that his wedding to Katie Holmes was in 2006. There is nothing in this to imply she is a Scientologist herself.

This is also a free text true or false Question. But it is also a *Value Judgement* question, because it asks you to make a qualitative assessment of the information when choosing an answer.

Value Judgement

Value Judgements can be introduced to any Item type.

Common examples:

- Which of the following best supports X?
- Which of the following is most/least likely to be true?
- Which of the following is the most influential cause of X?
- Which of these measures are most/least effective?
- Which of the following would strengthen/weaken X argument?
- When doing X, Y is… (e.g. good, bad, indifferent etc.).

Strategy:

1. Don't settle on an answer without assessing all options.

2. Dismiss non-viable answers and weigh up the remainder.

3. Go with best fit, even though there might be shades of grey.

Top Tip: Sometimes you will be asked about the *Author's View* on something in the passage. This is simply another way of introducing a Value Judgement, and the same rules apply.

Another Value Judgement you are often asked to make is whether something will *Strengthen or Weaken* the argument in the passage…

Educated Guessing

There is no negative marking. So, if in doubt: guess!

When guessing, go with your gut instinct. Your subconscious might have absorbed more than you realise. That nagging feeling in the back of your mind is often the result of genuine subconscious analysis.

If you really can't decide which option to go for, then choose 'Can't Tell'. Don't get bogged down on one statement.

> **Top Tip:** If you're stuck, guess and move on. Understanding the following clue words can help you to improve your odds by making 'educated guesses'.

Top Verbal Reasoning Tips

- Practice skimming passages for key words/phrases.
- Practice reading on a computer screen.
- Practice both Question Set formats.
- Recognise definitive or mitigating 'clue' words.
- Ask: 'Why has the question writer put these words in?'.
- Don't get stuck on one question – go with your gut instinct.
- Never use outside knowledge.
- Never assume causal relationships that aren't stated.
- Write your own questions to get in the mindset.

Time for some practice! Try answering the following 11 *Practice Sets*. Stick to the time limit of 22 minutes. Detailed explanations are provided. Good luck!

Practice Sets

Question 1

On 14 October 2012, 43-year-old Austrian Felix Baumgartner floated into space in a capsule suspended from a stratospheric balloon. When the balloon reached 128,000 feet, Felix jumped from the capsule's ledge towards the earth's surface. The time it took Felix to reach the ground after leaving the capsule was 9 minutes and 3 seconds. 4 minutes and 20 seconds of this time was spent in freefall. Felix reached a maximum velocity of 833.9 miles/hour.

The jump was almost aborted when Felix's helmet visor fogged up during his ascent into space. As he went through last-minute checks inside the capsule, it was found that a heater for his visor was not working. This meant the visor fogged up as he exhaled. 'This is very serious, Joe', he told retired US Air Force Col Joe Kittinger, whose records he was attempting to break, and who was acting as his radio link in mission control at Roswell airport.

Prior to Felix's jump, Kittinger held the records for highest, farthest, and longest freefall. These were set when he leapt from a helium envelope in 1960. Felix failed to break Kittinger's record for the longest freefall. After the jump, Felix thanked Kittinger for providing advice and encouragement throughout his preparation, and during the jump itself.

1. Felix returned to the Earth's surface 9 minutes and 3 seconds after leaving it in a stratospheric balloon

    A. True

    B. False

    C. Can't Tell

2. During his 1960 jump, Joe Kittinger was in freefall for more than 4 minutes and 20 seconds

    A. True

    B. False

    C. Can't Tell

3. Joe Kittinger reassured Felix via radio when his visor fogged up

    A. True

    B. False

    C. Can't Tell

4. Felix broke the sound barrier during his jump

    A. True

    B. False

    C. Can't Tell

Question 2

On 29 July 1908, Harland and Wolff presented the drawings for a proposed new ship to the Chairman of the White Star Line company, J. Bruce Ismay. These drawings were approved and work began on a truly vast vessel. The finished ship was 882 feet 6 inches long, and weighed 46,328 tonnes. Due to its unprecedented size, it was suggested that this ship should be called *Titanic*.

Shortly after 11.40 pm on 14 April 1912, this same ship hit an iceberg in the North Atlantic. This created a series of holes below the waterline. Four of the watertight compartments flooding might have been withstood. Five was too many. The ship sank, bow first, on 15 April 1912. There were only enough lifeboats to accommodate half of the people onboard. Had the ship been carrying its full capacity of 3,339, this would have been reduced to one third.

The wreck of the ship lies 12,000 feet below the ocean surface. It was found in 1985 by a Franco-American expedition. The team discovered that it had split apart, probably near or at the surface, before sinking to the seabed. Out of the 1,330 passengers and 870 crew who had been onboard, 1,500 died. After a 2004 expedition, photos were released of possible human remains on the ocean floor.

1. *Titanic* sunk on 15 April 1912

    A. True

    B. False

    C. Can't Tell

2. 700 people who had been on-board the ship survived

    A. True

    B. False

    C. Can't Tell

3. The ship would not have sunk if only four compartments had flooded

    A. True

    B. False

    C. Can't Tell

4. There were enough lifeboats to accommodate half the ship's capacity

    A. True

    B. False

    C. Can't Tell

Question 3

The richest man in history is J. D. Rockefeller. When he died in 1937, his estimated wealth, adjusted for the late 2000s, was between 392 and 664 billion US dollars. He was also the first person to accumulate personal wealth of $1 billion, passing that landmark in 1916. The source of Rockefeller's wealth was oil. His company, Standard Oil, which was established in Ohio in 1870, effectively came to hold a monopoly over oil supply in the US. In fact, it was ruled an illegal monopoly by the Supreme Court in 1911. Standard Oil's dominant position in the market was the result of Rockefeller's innovative strategies, which increased efficiency, combined with a ruthless approach to competing companies. After the Supreme Court ruling it was broken up into 33 subsidiaries, including ExxonMobil.

A good example of Standard Oil's ruthless strategy at work was the deals it made with the railroad companies. In 1868, the Lake Shore Railroad gave Rockefeller's firm a going rate of one cent a gallon or forty-two cents a barrel. This represented a 71% discount from its listed rates in return for a promise to ship at least 60 carloads of oil daily. The deal therefore dramatically increased Standard Oil's efficiency overnight. Then, in 1872, Rockefeller joined the South Improvement Company – a deal which paved the way for him to increase Standard Oil's efficiency once again by receiving rebates for shipping and drawbacks on oil his competitors shipped. When this deal became known, competitors convinced the Pennsylvania Legislature to revoke South Improvement's charter, however, and no oil was shipped under this arrangement.

The second richest man in history, Andrew Carnegie, also dealt in resources. He controlled the most extensive integrated iron and steel operations ever owned by an individual in the United States. Carnegie was the first person to use the Bessemer process on an industrial scale. This process removes impurities from iron by oxidation. The Carnegie Steel Company was sold to J. P. Morgan in 1901, leading to the creation of the US Steel Corporation. Carnegie's adjusted net worth was around $300 billion at the time of his death.

1. Rockefeller and Carnegie were both innovators

   A. True

   B. False

   C. Can't Tell

2. Rockefeller's wealth, adjusted for the late 2000s, passed $1 billion in 1916

   A. True

   B. False

   C. Can't Tell

3. Standard Oil's efficiency was increased by deals with the Lake Shore Railroad in 1868 and the South Improvement Company in 1872

   A. True

   B. False

   C. Can't Tell

4. ExxonMobil was created in 1911

   A. True

   B. False

   C. Can't Tell

Question 4

The two highest grossing movies of all time (not taking into account inflation) were both directed by James Cameron. His 2009 movie, *Avatar*, has taken more than any other film in history: $2.8 billion worldwide. Featuring the blue extra-terrestrials of the Na'vi tribe, who live on the habitable moon of Pandora, the 162-minute epic revolutionised the way 3D technology was used. At the centre of the plot is a romance between one of the Na'vi, Neytiri, and a human called Jake Sully. Sully has been sent to Pandora on behalf of a mining expedition to extract the valuable mineral, unobtainium. But when he and Neytiri fall in love, he ends up fighting for her tribe against his former employers.

Titanic is director Cameron's next highest-grossing film, taking $2.3 billion overall. The movie revolves around a romance between a blue-collar nomad called Jack Dawson and an aristocratic lady, Rose DeWitt Bukater. *Titanic* was first released in 1997. After it was re-released in 3D in April 2012, it took an additional $364 million, which is included in its overall gross takings. The movie was budgeted at $200 million and was the most expensive film ever made when it was released.

When the numbers are adjusted for inflation, the list of highest-grossing films looks different. *Avatar* drops to second place, and is trumped by *Gone with the Wind*. Since its release in 1939, the 220-minute epic has taken $3.3 billion. Two films directed by Steven Spielberg enter the top-ten highest-grossing films list when it is adjusted for inflation: *E.T. The Extra-Terrestrial* ($2.2 billion) and *Jaws* ($1.9 billion). *Titanic* falls to number four as it is overtaken by *Star Wars*.

1. *Avatar* and *Titanic* are the highest-grossing movies of all time (not taking into account inflation)

   A. True

   B. False

   C. Can't Tell

2. Steven Spielberg's two entries on the top-ten highest-grossing film list (adjusted for inflation) both feature non-human characters

   A. True

   B. False

   C. Can't Tell

3. Multiple James Cameron films feature romances between characters from different backgrounds

   A. True

   B. False

   C. Can't Tell

4. *Titanic* took more than $2 billion before April 2012

    A. True

    B. False

    C. Can't Tell

Question 5

The near-extinction of the dinosaurs occurred around 66 million years ago. We should say 'near-extinction', rather than 'extinction', since there are species of birds that are technically dinosaurs and live to this day. The technical name given to this 'near-extinction' is the 'Cretaceous–Paleogene extinction event' – or the 'K-Pg extinction event', for short. It marks the end of the Mesozoic Era and begins the Cenozoic Era. In the 1970s, palaeontologists started to come up with a variety of theories to explain the K-Pg event. There are fundamentally two schools of thought. One says that it was caused by an impact event, such as an asteroid collision. The other suggests that a confluence of various circumstances resulted in dinosaurs vanishing abruptly from the fossil records.

Within the fossil records, the time of the K-Pg extinction is marked by a thin layer of sediment known as the 'K-Pg boundary'. The boundary clay shows high levels of the metal iridium, which is rare in the Earth's crust but abundant in asteroids. This raises the possibility that the K-Pg event was caused by a giant asteroid or comet, which led to disturbances to the environment including the temporary shutdown of photosynthesis by land plants and plankton. The identification of the 110-mile-wide Chicxulub crater in Mexico provided conclusive evidence that the K-Pg boundary clay contained debris from an asteroid impact.

Among the other possible reasons for the K-Pg extinction, some palaeontologists point to climate change caused by decreasing volcanic activity. This would have cooled the earth significantly. Research proves that prior to the K-Pg extinction event, the Earth's poles had been 50 degrees centigrade hotter than they are today. Other scientists point to evidence of a significant drop in oxygen levels as the cause of the K-Pg extinction event. If large dinosaurs had respiratory systems similar to birds, this may have meant they become unable to fulfil the significant oxygen requirements of their bodies.

1. Which of the following can be logically inferred from the passage?

    A. There are two different theories put forward by palaeontologists to explain the K-Pg extinction event.

    B. Palaeontologists named the near extinction of the dinosaurs the Cretaceous–Paleogene extinction event.

    C. Palaeontologists did not come up with theories to explain the K-Pg extinction event prior to 1970.

    D. Palaeontologists only became aware of the K-Pg extinction event during the 1970s.

2. Which of the following statements, if true, would be most likely to weaken the argument that the K-Pg extinction event was caused by a comet or asteroid?

    A. The Chicxulub crater was re-measured and found to be only 100 miles wide, rather than 110 miles wide.

    B. High levels of iridium were found in fossil records from after the K-Pg extinction event.

C. Small traces of iridium found in fossil records from before the K-Pg extinction event.

D. The K-Pg boundary is found to relate to a different time period, much later than first thought.

3. The passage best supports which of the following statements?

   A. Climate change can lead to a decrease in volcanic activity.

   B. Large dinosaurs have similar respiratory systems to birds.

   C. The earth was hotter over 66 million years ago than it is today.

   D. Oxygen levels dropped dramatically before the K-Pg extinction event.

4. If the passage is true, which of the following is also true?

   A. The Cenozoic Era came before the Mesozoic Era.

   B. The Cenozoic Era followed the Mesozoic Era but not directly.

   C. There were no dinosaurs in the Cenozoic.

   D. The Mesozoic Era directly preceded the Cenozoic Era.

Question 6

One of the most important discoveries in the history of modern medicine happened in 1928, when the Scottish bacteriologist, Alexander Fleming, was studying influenza. One night, Fleming left open a culture dish containing the staphylococci germ. When Fleming returned in the morning, he discovered that a blue-green mould had formed in this dish, and that around this mould there was a bacteria-free circle, which looked like a small halo. Fleming named the active substance 'penicillin'.

However, it was Australian Howard Florey and Ernst Chain who developed penicillin so it could be produced as drug. Florey and Chain were awarded the Nobel Prize in 1945. Their advance allowed American drug companies to mass produce penicillin in the 1940s. In 1943, the best sample of the mould needed for penicillin production was found on a mouldy cantaloupe. One year later, in 1944, the USA produced 2.3 million doses of penicillin, most of which were ready in time for the invasion of Normandy. By mid-1945, 646 billion units were being produced per year in the USA, as a direct result of World War II.

1. World War II led to increased production of penicillin in the USA

   A. True

   B. False

   C. Can't Tell

2. Cantaloupes produce more of the mould needed to create penicillin than other fruits

   A. True

   B. False

   C. Can't Tell

3. Over 2 million doses of penicillin were used during the invasion of Normandy

   A. True

   B. False

   C. Can't Tell

4. Alexander Fleming discovered penicillin by accident

   A. True

   B. False

   C. Can't Tell

Question 7

The construction of the Eiffel Tower finished in 1889, and it served as the entrance to that year's World's Fair. It was, in 1889, the tallest building in the world, and remained so until the opening of the Chrysler Building in New York, 41 years later. The Eiffel Tower stands at 1,050 feet high (including an antenna that was added in 1957).

Work on the foundations of the Eiffel Tower started in January 1887. The actual iron work commenced after these were finished in June of that year. The 18,000 parts needed to construct the Eiffel Tower were detailed in 3,000 plan drawings. Many of the parts were riveted together in a factory in a Parisian suburb of Levallois-Perret and taken to the site of the Tower by horse and cart. The Eiffel Tower is made of iron. Obviously, iron rusts unless it is treated with chemicals, which can be found in certain types of paint. The Eiffel Tower is coated with 50–60 tonnes of paint every 7 years. Three different colours are typically used, in order to enhance the lighting effects on the tower.

In its long history, the Eiffel Tower has seen many interesting events and landmarks. Soon after its opening in September 1889, it was visited by Thomas Edison, who signed the guestbook. Upon the German occupation of Paris in 1940, the lift cables of the Tower were cut by the French so that Adolf Hitler would have to climb the steps. It was said that Hitler conquered France, but did not conquer the Eiffel Tower. On 28 November 2002, the Eiffel Tower received its 200 millionth guest.

1. The 1,050 feet Eiffel Tower was the world's tallest building in 1889

   A. True

   B. False

   C. Can't Tell

2. Thomas Edison and Adolf Hitler have visited the Eiffel Tower

   A. True

   B. False

   C. Can't Tell

3. Each plan drawing detailed six of the Eiffel Tower's parts

   A. True

   B. False

   C. Can't Tell

4. The Eiffel Tower is painted every 7 years to prevent rust

    A. True

    B. False

    C. Can't Tell

Question 8

Eddie Chapman was an English criminal who became a spy for the Nazis during World War II. He was known to the Germans by the codename *Fritz*. However, he defected back to his home country and worked for many years as a double agent for the British. Chapman had been imprisoned on the Channel Islands when they fell into German hands. From there he was transferred to a French jail, where he became acquainted with Captain Stephan von Gröning, head of the *Abwehr* in Paris. Chapman offered von Gröning his services as a turncoat agent.

After extensive training in explosives, radio communications and parachute jumping, Chapman was dropped into Cambridgeshire by the Germans on 16 December 1942. His mission was to sabotage the de Havilland aircraft factory in Hatfield. Instead, he surrendered to MI5. The sabotage was faked with their help in order to deceive the Germans. MI5 gave Eddie Chapman the codename *Zigzag* – a reference to the way he appeared to jump from one side to the other during the course of World War II.

By 1944, Chapman was sent back to Britain by the Germans in order to report on the accuracy of the coordinates they were programming into their V1 weapon. Chapman repeatedly reported back to the Germans that the bombs fired by the weapon were hitting Central London. In fact, they were falling well short. Through this misinformation, the British were able to ensure that the wrong coordinates continued to be used and that bombs from the V1 fell in the countryside rather than their target in the heart of the capital.

At the end of the war, Chapman received a £6,000 payment from MI5 and was allowed to keep £1,000 he had received from the Germans. He received no other money. He was granted a pardon for his pre-war activities. During the war, Chapman was also awarded the Iron Cross by the Germans for sabotaging the de Havilland aircraft factory.

1. Chapman received £7,000 at the end of the war

    A. True

    B. False

    C. Can't Tell

2. The V1 weapon was not accurate

    A. True

    B. False

    C. Can't Tell

3. Eddie Chapman, *Fritz* and *Zigzag* are the same person

    A. True

    B. False

    C. Can't Tell

4. The Germans were successfully deceived by a fake sabotage of the de Havilland aircraft factory

    A. True

    B. False

    C. Can't Tell

Question 9

One of the most prestigious awards that a fiction author can win is the Man Booker Prize for Fiction. Since its advent in 1969, it has been awarded every year for the best original full-length novel written in the English language by a citizen of the Commonwealth of Nations, Ireland or Zimbabwe. The prize money awarded with the Booker Prize was originally £21,000. It stayed the same until it was raised to £50,000 in 2002 after it was sponsored by the Man Group. It has remained at this level since then. This has made it one of the world's richest literary prizes.

From the time the prize was launched in 1969 until 2012, 23 of the winners have been from the UK. Hilary Mantel won in 2009 and 2012 with two sequential novels of the same genre. The winner in 2012 was the historical fiction book, *Bring up the Bodies*. Other authors who have won the Booker Prize more than once include Peter Carey, who triumphed in 1988 and 2001, and J. M. Coetzee, who took home the prize in 1983 and 1999.

In 1993, to mark the 25th anniversary of the Booker Prize, it was decided to choose a 'Booker of Bookers' Prize. Three previous judges of the award, Malcolm Bradbury, David Holloway and W. L. Webb chose *Midnight's Children* (the 1981 winner) as 'the best novel out of all the winners'. A similar prize, known as 'The Best of the Booker', was awarded in 2008 to celebrate the 40th anniversary of the Booker Prize. The winner, after a public vote, was once again Salman Rushdie's *Midnight's Children*.

1. The Man Group contributed an extra £29,000 to the prize money for the Booker Prize

    A. True

    B. False

    C. Can't Tell

2. The 2009 Booker Prize was won by a historical novel

    A. True

    B. False

    C. Can't Tell

3. Salmon Rushdie won the Booker Prize in 1981

   A. True

   B. False

   C. Can't Tell

4. Hilary Mantel has won £100,000 in prize money from the Booker Prize

   A. True

   B. False

   C. Can't Tell

Question 10

Robert Mugabe has been the leader of Zimbabwe for the three decades of its independence. He was a key figure in the struggle for independence, which involved a bitter bush war against a white minority that had cut the country loose from the colonial power Britain.

When he was first elected in 1980 he was praised for reaching out to the white minority and his political rivals, as well as for what was considered a pragmatic approach to the economy. However, he soon expelled from his government of national unity the party whose stronghold was in the south of the country and launched an anti-opposition campaign in which thousands died.

In the mid-1990s he embarked on a programme of land redistribution in which commercial farmers were driven off the land by mobs. The programme was accompanied by a steady decline in the economy. As the opposition to his rule increased, he and his ruling Zanu-PF party grew more determined to stay in power. Critics accuse him of heading a military regime.

In the elections of 2008, Zanu-PF lost its parliamentary majority and opposition leader Morgan Tsvangirai defeated Mr Mugabe in the presidential vote but with insufficient votes to avoid a run-off. Mr Mugabe was sworn in for another term in June 2008 after a widely condemned run-off vote from which Mr Tsvangirai withdrew because of attacks on his supporters. Because of international pressure, Mr Mugabe agreed a power-sharing deal with Mr Tsvangirai, who was made prime minister.

Adapted from http://www.bbc.co.uk/news/world-africa-14113249

1. Mugabe's land redistribution programme:

   A. Caused a negative impact on Zimbabwe's economy

   B. Took place in the early nineteen nineties

   C. Saw armed mobs drive commercial farmers off land

   D. Coincided with an economic downturn

2. Which of the following was not a consequence of the 2008 elections?

   A. Attacks on Mr Tsvangirai's supporters.

   B. Mugabe was made prime minister.

C. A run-off took place.

D. Mugabe was sworn in for another term.

3. Mugabe's approach to the economy:

   A. Was based on a programme of land distribution

   B. Was positively received at first

   C. Caused a steady decline

   D. Was likened by critics to that of a military regime

4. Which of the following can be inferred from the passage:

   A. Mugabe did not have much support in south Zimbabwe.

   B. Mugabe used violence to hold on to power.

   C. Mugabe is susceptible to international pressure.

   D. Mugabe was the main figure in Zimbabwe gaining independence.

Question 11

We all know how tempting it can be to have one too many chocolates or an extra slice of cake even when we know it would be healthier not to. But what drives this craving for sweet treats? Many scientists suggest that we are primed to desire sugar at an instinctive level as it plays such a vital role in our survival. Our sense of taste has evolved to covet the molecules vital to life like salt, fat and sugar.

When we eat food, the simple sugar glucose is absorbed from the intestines into the blood-stream and distributed to all cells of the body. Glucose is particularly important to the brain as it provides a major source of fuel to the billions of neuronal nerve cells. Neurons need a constant supply from the bloodstream as they don't have the ability to store glucose themselves. As diabetics know, someone with low blood sugar can quickly lapse into a coma.

According to the NHS, added sugars shouldn't make up more than 10% of the energy you get from food and drink each day. This is whether it comes from honey, fruit juice and jam, soft drinks, processed foods or table sugar. This works out at about 70 grams a day for men and 50 grams for women, although this can vary depending on your size, age and how active you are. Fifty grams of sugar is equivalent to 13 teaspoons of sugar a day, or two cans of fizzy drink, or eight chocolate biscuits.

When in the supermarket it's worth remembering that produce is classed as high in sugar if it contains more than 15 grams in 100 grams and low in sugar if it has less than 5 grams per 100 grams.

Adapted from http://www.bbc.co.uk/science/0/21835302

1. Which of the following statements is best supported by the passage?

   A. We are primed to desire sugar at an instinctive level.

   B. Added sugars shouldn't make up more than 10% of your daily energy.

   C. Low blood sugar levels can lead to a coma.

   D. All men should limit their added sugar intake to 70 grams of sugar per day.

2. Which of the following is not true?

    A. Glucose fuels neuronal nerve cells.

    B. 50 grams of sugar is equivalent to 13 teaspoons, 2 fizzy drinks and 8 chocolate biscuits.

    C. Produce with more than 15 grams in 100 grams is classed as high sugar in supermarkets.

    D. Neurons can't store glucose.

3. 50 grams of added sugar:

    A. Is the recommended daily intake, according to the NHS

    B. Is the ideal daily amount for every woman

    C. Is found in two fizzy drinks

    D. Is found in 8 chocolate biscuits

4. Which of the following can be a consequence of low blood sugar:

    A. Diabetes

    B. Sudden coma

    C. Fainting

    D. Death

Answers

Question 1

1. False

   We know from the first paragraph that it took Felix 9 minutes and 3 seconds to reach the earth 'after leaving the capsule'. However, we also know that he floated to 128,000 feet, suspended from a stratospheric balloon, before jumping from the capsule ledge. We can safely assume that this took some time. The answer, therefore, is 'False'.

2. True

   The key word is 'freefall'. We know from the first paragraph that Felix spent 4 minutes and 20 seconds in freefall. We know from the third paragraph that Joe Kittinger set the record for the longest freefall during his jump in 1960, and that Felix did not break this record. We can therefore infer that Kittinger was in freefall for longer than 4 minutes and 20 seconds.

3. Can't Tell

   We know from the second paragraph that Felix's visor fogged up. We know that he communicated this to Kittinger via radio. However, even though Felix did eventually jump, the passage does not say anywhere that Kittinger gave him any reassurance on this particular matter. Though the last paragraph refers to general 'advice and encouragement' given to Felix by Kittinger, this does not mean he reassured him about his visor fogging up.

4. Can't Tell

   We know that Felix reached a 'maximum velocity of 833.9 miles/hour'. However, the passage does not give the sound of speed. Nor does it state that Felix broke the sound barrier. You might personally know the speed of sound is 761.2 miles/hour. You might also have read in the news that Felix did, famously, break the sound barrier. But it is important that you do not bring outside knowledge into your reasoning. Based only on the information given in the passage, the answer is 'Can't Tell'.

Question 2

1. Can't Tell

   We know from the second paragraph that the ship described sank on 15 April 1912. But the only mention of the name *Titanic* is in the first paragraph: 'it was *suggested* that this ship should be called *Titanic*'. Although outside knowledge might tell us that this name was indeed adopted, using information in the passage alone we only know that the name *Titanic* was suggested. We do not know if this was the name that was actually given to the ship. Therefore, the answer is 'Can't Tell'.

2. True

   The last paragraph says: 'out of the 1,330 passengers and 870 crew onboard, 1,500 died'. We know from this that there were 1,330 + 870 = 2,200 people onboard. If 1,500 died, then 2,200 − 1,500 = 700 survived.

3. Can't Tell

The key word is 'compartments'. Paragraph two says: 'four of the watertight compartments flooding might have been withstood'. The word 'might' tells us that we do not know for sure whether four compartments flooding would have sunk the ship. Therefore, the answer is 'Can't Tell'.

4. False

From the end of the second paragraph, we know that: 'there were only enough lifeboats to accommodate half of the people *onboard*'. But we are interested in how many of its *capacity* the lifeboats could accommodate. The next sentence says: 'had the ship been carrying its full capacity of 3,339, this would have been reduced to one third'. Therefore, there were only enough lifeboats to carry one third, rather than one half, of the ship's capacity.

Question 3

1. True

Searching for the word 'innovator' or its derivatives leads us to a sentence towards the end of the first paragraph: 'Standard Oil's dominant position in the market was the result of *Rockefeller's innovative strategies*'. We can infer from this that Rockefeller was an innovator. For information on Carnegie, we must look in the final paragraph. Though the word 'innovator' is not used, we should take note of the word 'first', since being the first to do something logically infers innovation. As 'Carnegie was *the first person* to use the Bessemer process on an industrial scale', we can therefore confirm that we was an innovator as well. So the answer is 'True'.

2. False

Searching for key words leads us to the third sentence in the first paragraph, which tells us that Rockefeller was 'the first person to accumulate personal wealth of $1 billion, passing that landmark in 1916'. But for him to pass that landmark in 1916, that must have been his actual wealth in 1916 – not adjusted for the late 2000s. Though the previous sentence states that his overall wealth of 'between 392 and 664 billion US dollars' is adjusted in this way, it is illogical to apply this caveat to the figure of $1 billion as well.

3. False

The relevant information is in the second paragraph. We can quickly see that the 1868 deal with the Lakeshore Railroad 'increased Standard Oil's efficiency overnight'. We also know that the 1872 deal with the South Improvement Company 'paved the way for him [Rockefeller] to increase Standard Oil's efficiency once again'. However, reading on a little further, we see that, after protests, 'no oil was shipped under this arrangement'. Therefore, efficiency was only increased by the Lake Shore Railroad deal in 1968, and *not* by the 1872 deal with the South Improvement company. The answer is therefore 'False'.

4. Can't Tell

Scanning for 'ExxonMobil' and '1911' takes us to two sentences in the first paragraph. One tells us that Standard Oil was ruled to be an illegal monopoly by the Supreme

Court in 1911. The other tells us that after the Supreme Court ruling, Standard Oil was 'broken up into 33 subsidiaries, including ExxonMobil'. But since it is not stated exactly how long after the ruling the company was broken up, we 'Can't Tell' when ExxonMobil was created.

Question 4

1. True

    Looking for the first key words – 'highest-grossing movies of all time (not taking into account inflation)' – leads us straight to the first line, where we read that the top two were both directed by James Cameron. The next sentence gives more relevant information, saying that 'his' film, 'Avatar', our next key word, 'has taken more than any other film in history'. This is the same as saying that it is the highest-grossing film of all time (before inflation). Our next key word is 'Titanic', and we first see this at the start of the second paragraph where we are told: 'Cameron's next highest-grossing film, taking $2.3 billion'. Since we know that Cameron directed the two highest-grossing films of all time and we know that Avatar was the highest-grossing film of all time, we can infer that if Titanic was Cameron's second-highest grossing film, it was also the second-highest grossing film of all time. So the answer is 'True'.

2. Can't Tell

    Searching for mention of 'Spielberg' takes us to the end of the third paragraph. We can verify from this that: 'two films directed by Steven Spielberg enter the top-ten highest-grossing films list when it is adjusted for inflation'. We are also told that these are titled E.T. The Extra-Terrestrial and Jaws. However, we are told nothing in the passage about the content of these films, so we have no idea if they feature 'non-human characters'. Remember not to bring in outside knowledge! It is also not true to say that the film title E.T. The Extra-Terrestrial logically infers the presence of a 'non-human character' since film titles are not necessarily descriptive. (e.g. Reservoir Dogs contains neither dogs, nor a reservoir). Even if it did, however, Jaws could refer to anything in this context.

3. True

    We need to look for the key word 'romance'. In the first paragraph, this will tell us that in Cameron's Avatar 'the centre of the plot is a romance between one of the Na'vi, Neytiri and a human called Jake Sully'. This certainly classifies as a romance between charac-ters from different backgrounds. But in order to verify the statement, we need to know if this is the case in 'multiple' Cameron films – more than one. Continuing to look for the key word 'romance' we get to the second paragraph. Here we are told that Cameron's Titanic 'revolves around a romance between a blue-collar nomad called Jack Dawson and an aristocratic lady, Rose DeWitt Bukater'. This also fits the description of a romance between characters from different backgrounds. The answer is therefore 'True'.

4. False

    We are looking for figures relating to Titanic. This takes us only to the second paragraph. We know from the first sentence that the movie took $2.3 billion. But if we look for the key words 'April 2012', we learn that this number includes $364 million taken after the film was re-released in 3D on that date. Since $2.3 billion – $364 million is less than $2 billion, the film cannot have taken more than $2 billion before that date. The answer is therefore 'False'.

Question 5

1. C

   Locating the key word '1970s' leads us to the line: 'In the 1970s, palaeontologists started to come up with a variety of theories to explain the K-Pg extinction event'. The word 'started' logically infers that this had not happened before the 1970s, which began in 1970. None of the other statements can be logically inferred from the passage:

   A. Though we are told that there a 'fundamentally two schools of thought', in this context 'fundamentally' acts as a mitigating term, meaning 'broadly speaking' or 'for the most part'. The preceding sentence also tells us explicitly that there are 'a variety of theories'. Some of these are even highlighted in the final paragraph.

   B. Though we are told that Cretaceous–Paleogene extinction event was 'the technical name given' to the near extinction of the dinosaurs, we do not know if it was given by palaeontologists.

   D. We know that palaeontologists 'started to come up with a variety of theories' to explain the K-Pg event in the 1970s, but this is not the same as saying they only became aware of it in the 1970s.

2. D

   In order to get the answer we need to go through each statement, one by one. Our thought process for each statement should work as follows:

   A. This is a clear decoy. There is no evidence that altering the measurement of the Chicxulub crater by less than 10% would have any impact on the asteroid/comet theory.

   B. This might suggest another asteroid after the K-Pg extinction event, but this would not make it less likely that one caused the K-Pg extinction event in the first place.

   C. 'Small traces' of iridium is consistent with the fact that the passage tells us that iridium is 'rare' in the Earth's crust. Had there been high levels of iridium prior to the K-Pg extinction event, we might have inferred that there was another asteroid prior to the K-Pg extinction event that the dinosaurs survived, which could have weakened the argument.

   D. The theory of the asteroid or comet causing the K-Pg extinction event is heavily reliant on the high levels of iridium found in the K-Pg boundary. If this layer of sediment in fact related to a later time period significantly after the K-Pg extinction event, this would therefore significantly weaken the argument.

3. C

   In order to get the answer we need to go through each statement, one by one. Our thought process for each statement should work as follows:

   A. Reference to climate change and volcanic activity leads us to the start of the final paragraph, where we are told that some people cite 'climate change caused by decreasing volcanic activity' as a reason for the K-Pg extinction event. This is, in fact, directly opposed to the statement, which suggests it is climate change that can lead to a decrease in volcanic activity, rather than vice-versa.

B. Looking for key terms takes us to the last sentence, where we are told that 'if large dinosaurs had respiratory systems similar to birds' it might support theories about a drop in oxygen levels leading to the K-Pg extinction event. 'If' is a clear mitigation, and suggests the statement is speculative – we do not know if large dinosaurs did in fact have respiratory systems similar to birds.

C. The information in this statement is split across the passage. Reference to '66 million years ago' takes us to the first paragraph, where we learn that this was approximately when the K-Pg extinction event occurred. Reference to the temperature of the earth leads us to the final paragraph, where we are told that before the K-Pg extinction event, 'the Earth's poles had been 50 degrees centigrade hotter than they are today'. Linking these two pieces of information means that the passage therefore supports the assertion that the Earth was hotter over 66 million years ago than it is today.

D. Should we need to check the final statement, we would learn from the passage that 'some scientists point to evidence of a significant drop in oxygen levels'. The fact that there is evidence of a significant drop in oxygen levels, and that some scientists point to this, is not the same as saying there *was* a significant drop in oxygen levels. So while this could be true, it is less likely than option C.

4. D

The words 'Mesozoic and 'Cenozoic' occur in the first paragraph, where we are told that the K-Pg extinction event 'marks the end of the Mesozoic Era and begins the Cenozoic Era'. Since the word 'preceded' means 'comes before', this confirms that the Mesozoic Era 'preceded' the Cenozoic Era. And since the same event marked the end of the Mesozoic and the start of the Cenozoic Era, we can also verify that it preceded it 'directly'. The other statements are all false or uncertain:

A. For the aforementioned reasons, we know that the Mesozoic Era came before the Cenozoic Era, rather than vice-versa.

B. It is true that the Cenozoic Era followed the Mesozoic Era, but for the above-mentioned reasons we know that it did follow directly.

C. Though the Cenozoic Era followed the K-Pg extinction event, we know that this marked the 'near extinction', rather than the full extinction, of the dinosaurs.

Question 6

1. True

'World War II' is the last phrase of the entire passage. Scanning the preceding sentences for context, we learn that: 'in 1944, the USA produced 2.3 million doses of penicillin', that 'by mid-1945, 646 billion units were being produced per year in the USA' and that this was 'as a direct result of World War II'. The fact that penicillin production in the USA went from 2.3 million units in 1944 to 646 billion units in 1945 shows that production did increase. The fact that this happened 'as a *direct result* of World War II' verifies that it was, indeed, World War II that led to this increased production. So the answer is 'True'.

2. Can't Tell

'Cantaloupe' is a nice key word, as it stands out as quite unusual. When we locate it in the passage, we are told that 'in 1943, the best sample of the mould needed for penicillin production was found on a mouldy cantaloupe'. But all this tells us is that in one particular year, the best sample of the mould needed for penicillin that was actually found, happened to be on a cantaloupe. The one-year time frame and the fact that it was only the best mould 'found', rather than the best mould per se, both tell us that this was a specific case. Moreover, there is no context given about other fruits. We cannot, therefore, logically extrapolate from this one-off example a long-term trend whereby cantaloupes produce more of the mould in question than other fruits. Nor can we rule it out. So we 'Can't Tell'.

3. Can't Tell

Another good key word, as it only arises once in the passage, is 'Normandy'. In context, we see that: 'the USA produced 2.3 million doses of penicillin, most of which was ready in time for the invasion of Normandy'. But this only tells us roughly how much penicillin was produced in time for Normandy. It does not logically infer anything about how much was used there.

4. Can't Tell

Fleming and his role in the discovery of penicillin are cited in the early part of the passage. The key line is: 'Fleming left open a culture dish containing the staphylococci germ', as this is what led to the creation of the mould which he christened 'penicillin'. However, there is nothing within the passage to tell us whether the culture dish was left open on purpose or by mistake. Remember not to bring in outside knowledge here. Based on the information available, the answer is 'Can't Tell'.

Question 7

1. False

We can verify in the first paragraph that the Eiffel Tower 'was, in 1889, the tallest building in the world'. Scanning for the given measurement, we can also see that it stands at 1,050 feet high. However, we are also told, in the parentheses, that this measurement is 'including an antenna that was added in 1957'. We can therefore infer that before 1957, the Eiffel Tower was less than 1,050 feet tall. So while it was the world's tallest building in 1889, it was not then 1,050 feet tall. The answer is therefore 'False'.

2. Can't Tell

The key reference points are 'Thomas Edison' and 'Adolf Hitler' – both mentioned in the final paragraph. We are told categorically that 'in September 1889, [the Eiffel Tower] was visited by Thomas Edison'. So that part of the statement is verified. In terms of Hitler, we can read that: 'the lift cables of the Tower were cut by the French so that Adolf Hitler would have to climb the steps'. However, this refers to a hypothetical situation – if Hitler visited. There is nothing to tell us whether he actually did or didn't. The phrase: 'It was said that Hitler conquered France, but did not conquer the Eiffel Tower', sheds no further light on this matter. And thus we 'Can't Tell'.

3. Can't Tell

   We should scan the passage for the term 'plan drawing', and in particular the number of parts included in each of these. In the second paragraph, one sentence tells us that: 'The 18,000 parts needed to construct the Eiffel Tower were detailed in 3,000 plan drawings'. If each plan drawing detailed an equal number of parts, we could infer that each one detailed six parts. Since this is not stated or inferred, however, we cannot make this assumption. However, the possibility is not discounted, either. So the answer is 'Can't Tell'.

4. Can't Tell

   We know from the end of the second paragraph, having looked for our key phrases, that: 'the Eiffel Tower is coated with 50–60 tonnes of paint every 7 years'. Looking for reference to 'rust' takes us to the preceding sentence, where we are told that: 'iron rusts, unless it is treated with chemicals, which can be found in certain types of paint'. So the passage confirms two things: (1) the Eiffel Tower is painted every 7 years, and (2) some paints contain anti-rust chemicals. But the passage does not logically infer that the paint used on the Eiffel Tower is in fact the type that does contain anti-rust chemicals, or that the purpose of the 7-yearly painting is to prevent rust. The statements are juxtaposed, but not necessarily directly related, unless by assumption, which is to be avoided. So the answer is 'Can't Tell'.

Question 8

1. False

   The appropriate figures are located in the final paragraph. First, we are told that 'at the end of the war, Chapman received a £6,000 payment from MI5'. From this alone, we know that he received *at least* £6,000 at the end of the war. Then we read that he 'was allowed to keep £1,000 he had received from the Germans'. However, the fact that he was 'keeping' £1,000 that 'he had received' (past tense) infers that this was received *before* the end of the war. As the next sentence confirms that Chapman 'received no other money', we know that he *received* only £6,000 at the end of the war – even though he *kept* £1,000 he already had. So it is 'False' to say he received £7,000.

2. Can't Tell

   Straight away, we search for any references to the 'V1 weapon'. At the start of the second paragraph, we learn that: 'Chapman was sent back to Britain by the Germans, in order to report on the accuracy of the coordinates they were programming into their V1 weapon'. This tells us that the V1 weapon depends on the accuracy of the coordinates that are put into it. We also know that Chapman reported to the Germans that bombs fired by the weapon were hitting Central London, even though 'they were falling well short'. But the only definitive reason given for the bombs falling short of their Central London 'target' is the 'misinformation' given by the British, which ensured that the Germans continued using the 'wrong coordinates'. Had the right coordinates been used, we do not know whether the weapon would have proved accurate or not, so the answer is 'Can't Tell'.

3. True

   'Fritz' is mentioned in the second sentence of the first paragraph, which confirms that this was the name that the Germans had for Eddie Chapman: 'Eddie Chapman was an English criminal, who became a spy for the Nazis during the Second World War. He was known to the Germans by the codename Fritz'. So we know that 'Chapman' and 'Fritz' are the same person. When we find the name 'Zigzag' in the second paragraph, we see that: 'MI5 gave Eddie Chapman the codename Zigzag'. Piecing this together, we know that Fritz = Chapman = Zigzag. So the answer is 'True'.

4. True

   The 'de Havilland aircraft factory' is mentioned twice. The first time is in the second paragraph. Here we learn that the sabotage of the factory was 'was faked with [MI5's] help, in order to deceive the Germans'. But we do not know from this part of the passage whether the Germans were *successfully* deceived or not. However, looking at the second mention of the 'de Havilland aircraft factory' in the last sentence of the passage, we see that: 'Chapman was also awarded the Iron Cross by the Germans for sabotaging the de Havilland aircraft factory'. The fact that the Germans acted on the basis that Chapman had sabotaged the factory infers that they believed that this was the case. Thus, the sabotage did *successfully* deceive them and the answer is 'True'.

Question 9

1. Can't Tell

   Skimming for 'prize money' and 'Man Group' takes us to midway through the first paragraph: 'The prize money awarded with the Booker Prize was originally £21,000. It stayed the same until it was raised to £50,000 in 2002, after it was sponsored by the Man Group'. From this we know two things: (1) the prize money went up by £29,000, and (2) that this happened in 2002, after the Booker was sponsored by the Man Group. Since the Man Group were sponsoring the Booker Prize, it might be fair to assume that they contributed some money towards it. But we do not know that this went directly towards prize money. And, even if it did, we do not know that this contribution alone accounted for the entire £29,000 increase. Nor is there anything to suggest this wasn't the case. Hence, we 'Can't Tell'.

2. True

   A quick search for '2009' tells us that: 'Hilary Mantel won in 2009 and 2012, with two sequential novels of the same genre'. So we know that Mantel won in 2009 and that the book was the same genre as the winner in 2012. Therefore, even though the genre of the 2009 winner is not stated directly, we can find out more if we know the genre of the 2012 winner. The next sentence says: 'The winner in 2012 was the *historical fiction* book, *Bring up the Bodies*'. Since the 2009 and 2012 winners were books of the same genre, we can infer that the 2009 winner was also 'historical fiction', making the statement 'True'.

3. True

   Searching for '1981', we see that '[...] Webb chose *Midnight's Children* (the 1981 winner) [...]'. So we know that the 1981 Booker Prize winner was *Midnight's Children*. If we look no further, we might be tempted to go for 'Can't Tell', since this part of the passage does not tell us that Salman Rushdie wrote *Midnight's Children*. But if we are also skimming for the key words 'Salman Rushdie', then we come to the last line, which refers to 'Salman Rushdie's *Midnight's Children*'. This tells us that Salman Rushdie is the author of *Midnight's Children*. Putting these two pieces of information together, we know that *Midnight's Children* won in 1981 and that it was written by Salman Rushdie. Therefore, Salman Rushdie did win the Booker in 1981 and the answer is 'True'.

4. Can't Tell

There are two relevant pieces of information, both of which have formed parts of previous statements, which should save us time. The first is about prize money, and we know that the prize money 'was raised to £50,000 in 2002, after it was sponsored by the Man Group. It has remained at this level since then'. The second relevant statement says that: 'Hilary Mantel won in 2009 and 2012'. From this information, we know that Hilary Mantel won £50,000 in 2009 and £50,000 in 2012. This alone equals £100,000 in prize money. However, though we are told that Mantel won in 2009 and 2012, we are not told that these were the *only* times she won. Therefore, she might have won the Booker on more occasions and received more prize money, bringing the total above £100,000. So we 'Can't Tell' if she has won £100,000 or if she has won more.

Question 10

1. D

We are told in the third paragraph that 'The [land redistribution] programme was accompanied by a steady decline in the economy'. 'Accompanied' can mean 'happened at the same time as', and a 'steady decline in the economy' fits with 'economic downturn'. Therefore, it is accurate to say that the programme 'coincided with an economic downturn'.

  A. Though we know that the programme was 'accompanied by economic decline', we do not know that the programme was the cause of that decline. Be careful not to assume cause and effect!

  B. The passage clearly says that the programme took place in the mid-, rather than 'early-', 1990s.

  C. We know that 'mobs' drove commercial farmers off the land. However, there is no evidence that these mobs were 'armed'.

2. B

The final paragraph says that 'Mr Tsvangirai was made prime minister' as part of a power sharing regime. Though Mugabe was earlier 'sworn in', we do not know in what capacity.

  A. The previous sentence says that Mr Tsvangirai withdrew from the run-off because of attacks on his supporters.

  C. There are two references to this run-off in the final paragraph.

  D. As per B, we are told that 'Mugabe was sworn in for another term'.

3. B

The second paragraph says of Mugabe: 'When he was first elected in 1980 he was praised for reaching out to the white minority and his political rivals, *as well as for what was considered a pragmatic approach to the economy'*. Since he was praised for his pragmatic approach to the economy, and this praise came when he was first elected, we can fairly conclude that his economic approach was received positively at first.

A. Though we know this programme was implemented in the mid-1990s, there is no evidence that it was what Mugabe's economic approach was 'based on'.

C. We know there was a 'steady decline in the economy' but we cannot automatically conclude that this was a result of Mugabe's economic approach, since this is not stated. Economic decline can have a number of causes not related to the government's economic approach – for example, natural disaster.

D. Though critics did liken Mugabe's to a 'military regime', nowhere was this linked to economic policy.

4. C

In the final paragraph, we are told that 'Because of international pressure, Mr Mugabe agreed a power-sharing deal with Mr Tsvangirai, who was made prime minister'. So, we know that there was international pressure, and we know that Mugabe acted 'because of this' – 'because of' being the key bridging phrase.

A. Though we know from the second paragraph that 'he soon expelled from his government of national unity the party whose stronghold was in the south', this is not the same as saying Mugabe lacked support in the South.

B. There is nothing specifically stating this. Though there is some reference to violence, and a clear reference to the fact that 'he and his ruling Zanu-PF party grew more determined to stay in power', the two things are never explicitly linked with a clear bridging phrase.

D. We know from the first paragraph that Mugabe was 'a key figure in the struggle for independence'. However, being '*a*' key figure implies there were others, so saying he was '*the*' key figure is not accurate based on the information given.

Question 11

1. C

The end of the second paragraph says: 'As diabetics know, someone with low blood sugar can quickly lapse into a coma'. The use of the word 'know' is key as it supports the fact that what follows is factually correct. And indeed, the information about people with low blood sugar potentially lapsing into comas is presented in definitive terms – unlike any of the other answer options.

A. We are told in the first paragraph that 'Many scientists suggest' this is the case. That does not mean that it definitely is the case. Since it is less definitive than option C, it is not, therefore, the best supported statement.

B. The third paragraph effectively says this, but the information is introduced with the caveat: 'According to the NHS'. Again, this means it is subjective rather than objective, unlike option C.

D. Again, this follows from the NHS opinion, and is therefore subjective. Furthermore, the amount of added sugar will 'vary depending on your size, age and how active you are'. So 70 grams will not be an accurate figure for 'all men'.

2. B

This statement is false because of one word: 'and'. The passage says, at the end of the penultimate paragraph, that 50 grams of sugar is equivalent to: '13 teaspoons of sugar a day, *or* two cans of fizzy drink, *or* eight chocolate biscuits'. It is possible to miss this detail when scanning quickly, so make sure you hone in on relevant parts of the passage and pick up the requisite level of detail.

A. The second paragraph confirms that glucose is a 'major source of fuel to the billions of neuronal nerve cells'.

C. The final sentence confirms that 'produce is classed as high in sugar if it contains more than 15 grams in 100 grams'.

D. The second paragraph confirms that 'Neurons need a constant supply from the bloodstream as they don't have the ability to store glucose themselves'.

3. D

The last sentence of the third paragraph says that 'fifty grams of sugar is equivalent to ... eight chocolate biscuits'. 'Equivalent to' in this context – referring to sugar content – means that 50 grams of sugar is found in 8 chocolate biscuits. The full statement – '50 grams of sugar is found in 8 chocolate biscuits' – would therefore be 'True'.

A. The third paragraph gives 50 grams as the daily recommended intake specifically for women. The recommended daily intake for men is 70 grams. Therefore, this is an over-generalisation and consequently 'False'.

B. Once again, we must take note of the fact that, though the recommended daily amount for women is 50 grams per day, this will 'vary depending on your size, age and how active you are'. So 50 grams cannot logically be said to be ideal for 'every' woman.

C. By the same logic that makes 'D' the correct answer, we know that 50 grams of sugar is found in 'two cans of fizzy drink'. On the face of it, the complete statement – '50 grams of sugar is found in 2 fizzy drinks' – therefore appears to be 'True'. However, the passage specifies that 50 grams of sugar is equivalent to two '*cans of*' fizzy drink. Therefore, the valid response to the full statement would actually be 'Can't Tell' rather than 'True'. If the two fizzy drinks were in cans, then yes, it would be 'True'. But if they were in big, 2-litre bottles, then the answer would be 'False'. We don't know.

4. B

The last sentence of the second paragraph says: 'As diabetics know, someone with low blood sugar can quickly lapse into a coma'. If it had said that 'diabetics think...' or 'diabetics believe...' then we would not be able to tell if what followed was a genuine consequence. However, the verb 'know' is definitive and therefore what follows must be 'True'. The use of the word 'sudden' in the answer is borne out by the use of the word '*quickly*' in the passage.

A. There is nothing to support this in the passage alone. Though diabetics know the consequences of low blood sugar, this does not logically affirm that diabetes is a consequence of low blood sugar.

C. There is no mention of this, and this answer would require an assumption.

D. There is no mention of this, and this answer would require an assumption.

CHAPTER 2

Decision Making

Overview

The Decision Making section of the UKCAT is the latest addition to the exam. It replaced Decision Analysis, a section previously designed to assess logic and decision making during times of uncertainty. In some respects, the new Decision Making section combines certain elements of both Quantitative and Verbal Reasoning.

The Decision Making section is designed to test a number of skills, including deductive reasoning, evaluating arguments and statistical reasoning. When first launched in 2017, students performed well in this section, with an average score of 647.

Format of the Section

You will be faced with 29 questions to be answered in 32 minutes (including 1 minute of reading time). This gives just over 64 seconds per question. Each question contains text and may contain additional information in the form of tables, charts, graphs or diagrams. Unlike other sections, each question is a standalone question, so you will be faced with 29 different sets of information to interpret.

When we analyse the section further, we can break down the types of question in more detail:

- Recognising assumptions
- Interpreting information and drawing conclusions

  Evaluating arguments
  35%: 10–11 Qs

- Logical puzzles
- Syllogisms

  Deductive reasoning
  35%: 10–11 Qs

- Venn diagrams
- Probabilistic and statistical reasoning

  Statistical and figural reasoning
  30%: 8–9 Qs

Evaluating arguments constitutes approximately 35% of the exam, or 10–11 questions. Within this category of question you will need to understand how to identify an assumption within an argument, as well as how to correctly interpret information and draw conclusions. This might involve a mixture of text and graphical information. Deductive reasoning forms another 35% of the section, with questions in the form of logical puzzles and syllogisms. The remaining 30% of questions involve statistical and figural reasoning – using Venn diagrams and basic probability and statistics to answer questions. You will have access to the on-screen calculator throughout this section.

> **Top Tip:** Although the UKCAT is an aptitude test, having a solid grasp of critical thinking and probability will certainly help you through this section. !

Decision Making Layout

The question layout is slightly different in this section as compared to other sections. For the majority of questions, the information will be displayed with the questions beneath, as illustrated in the following diagram:

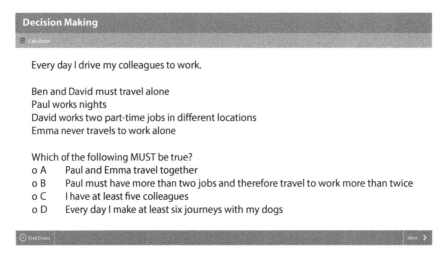

For these questions you simply need to click on your chosen answer, then 'Next'. Typically, there will be four options to choose from. A second type of question format is the 'drag-and-drop' style question. In these questions you will be presented with information followed by five statements. Next to each statement you will need to place either a 'Yes' or 'No', as shown in the following:

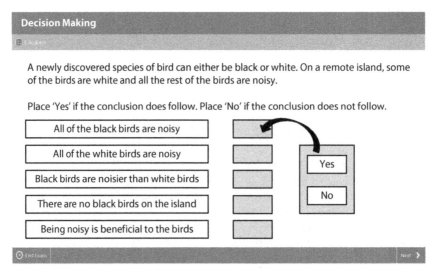

These five-part questions do not however score five marks! Instead, you need to get all five stems correct to score two marks, or four stems correct to score one mark. Three or less scores you 0!

Top Tip: Some of the questions can be tricky to do on a computer – use your pen and notebook to make diagrams and perform calculations.

Evaluating Arguments

Before we begin looking at assumptions and conclusions, let's look at the fundamentals of an argument. An argument can be defined as a set of reasons given in support of an idea. As such, arguments contain two crucial components: premise(s) and conclusion(s).

A premise can simply be thought of as the evidence or reasons given in support of the conclusion. From the given premise(s), conclusions can follow. A conclusion is therefore the proposition reached from the given premise(s).

To simplify this, imagine your argument is the Parthenon in Greece. Just like the roof of the Parthenon is held up by the pillars, the conclusion is supported by the premises. The greater the number of and the more substantial the premises, the more solid the conclusion will be.

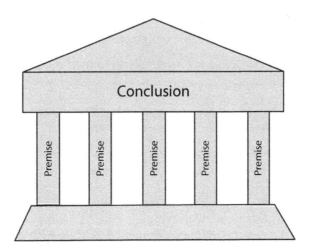

Assumptions

An assumption can be defined as something which is accepted as true or certain to happen, but without evidence. It can therefore be thought of as a premise that is not stated within the argument. Or, as a see-through pillar in the Parthenon model.

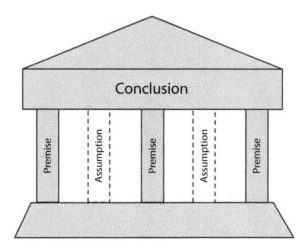

The more assumptions that are present in the argument, the weaker it becomes.

Let's look at a practice question. Take 60 seconds to answer *Example Question 1*. Make a note of your answer before moving on to the explanation.

Example Question 1

Should the government increase the daily recommended fruit and vegetable intake from five to seven portions a day?

Select the strongest argument from the following statements:

A. Yes, evidence shows that there are fewer health concerns if you regularly eat fruit and vegetables.

B. Yes, healthier snacks in general will improve life expectancy.

C. No, an extra two recommended fruits per day may be too expensive for some people.

D. No, people who take seven fruits and vegetable portions a day have been shown to have little differences in health compared to those who take five fruit and vegetable portions a day.

Approaching Assumption Based Questions

This was an example of an assumption based question, combining various factors which may strengthen or weaken an argument.

In order to form a strong argument, the premises should

- Directly connect to the subject matter.
- Be objective.
- Be evidence based.

The main factors which will weaken a premise are:

- Vague or no link to the conclusion
- Contain subjective opinions
- Rely on assumptions

Just as in Verbal Reasoning, it's therefore important to pay close attention to the choice of wording. Definitive words such as must, always and never will form strong arguments, whereas mitigating words such as sometimes or some will form much weaker arguments.

Example Question 1: Answer and Explanation

Statement A: Although evidence based, there is no quantifiable number of how many fruit/vegetables leads to 'fewer health concerns', compared to option D. What defines 'regular'? You would need to make various assumptions to justify this option.

Statement B: Fruits and vegetables are of course a type of healthy snack. However, the question does not focus on healthier snacks but specifically fruit and vegetables. This is an example of where the premise is not directly related to the conclusion.

Statement C: This does not focus on both fruits and vegetables, only fruits.

Statement D: A clear evidence basis showing no reason to increase from five to seven fruits or vegetables per day.

Interpreting Information and Drawing Conclusions

We have already looked at conclusions in the Verbal Reasoning section of this book, however, conclusion based questions may also appear in Decision Making. Remember, a conclusion is one that *logically follows* from the information.

In Decision Making, drawing conclusions can be combined with interpreting information. Data may be presented in numerous forms, including graphs, tables, charts and diagrams. Often, you will need to combine the information presented with some written information in order to draw a conclusion.

Let's look at a practice question. Take 60 seconds to answer *Example Question 2*. Make a note of your answer before moving on to the explanation.

Example Question 2

The student committee made a map with the layout for the location of the stalls in the sports hall for the student fair.

The knitting society was located as far as possible from the jazz club.

The rock climbing society is equidistant from the tennis club and the photography group.

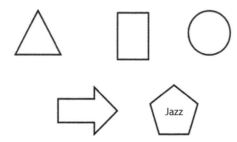

Which of the following must be true?

    A. The arrow is the tennis club.

    B. The rectangle is the rock climbing society.

    C. The circle is the photography group.

    D. The arrow is the knitting society.

Example Question 2: Answer and Explanation

This is an example of a diagram based question. Some students struggle with keeping several 'rules' or premises in their min whilst applying logic, in which case it makes sense to quickly draw a visual representation in your laminated notebook. This will then allow you to quickly make annotations as you look at each premise in turn. By applying the known facts we can draw the following:

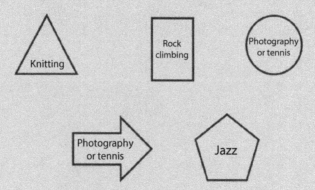

Statements A and C may not be true as we cannot determine which out of the circle and arrow, the photography group and tennis are represented by.

Statement D is incorrect as if the knitting society was represented by the arrow, it would not be located as far as possible from the jazz club.

This leaves us with Statement B as the only option which must be true.

Deductive Reasoning

Deductive reasoning is a logical process in which a conclusion is based on the concordance of multiple premises that are generally assumed to be true. In other words, in deductive reasoning, you will be presented with a number of rules that apply to a general principle, then be expected to apply those rules to a specific scenario.

In Decision Making, the two types of deductive reasoning questions are syllogisms and logical puzzles.

Approaching Syllogisms

Syllogisms are a form of reasoning where a conclusion is reached from two or more given premises. A common term will be present in the premises but not the conclusion. These question formats lend themselves nicely to the 'drag-and-drop' style of questions.

An example of a syllogism is the statement:

All humans are mammals. All mammals are warm blooded. Therefore, all humans are warm blooded.

To help simplify this, we can put the argument into letter format:

All A = B

All B = C

Therefore, A = C

Let's look at a practice question. Take 60 seconds to answer *Example Question 3*. Make a note of your answer before moving on to the explanation.

Example Question 3

> Everyone in the class can swim, except for Molly and Jeremy. More than three people in the class can ride a bike.

Place 'Yes' if the conclusion does follow. Place 'No' if the conclusion does not follow.

    A. At least three people in the class can swim.

    B. Molly and Jeremy must be able to ride a bike.

    C. There are more people who can swim than there are people who can ride a bike.

    D. If Molly can ride a bike, Jeremy must also be able to ride a bike.

    E. There are more people who can swim than there are people who cannot swim.

Example Question 3: Answer and Explanation

In this question there are two premises provided. For each statement you need to see whether a conclusion logically follows or not.

Remember that in drag-and-drop questions you need to score all five statements correct to score 2 marks, and four correct to score 1 mark.

Statement A: No

As 'more than three people' in the class can ride a bike, this means that there are at least four people in the class. If we take into account that Molly and Jeremy cannot swim, this means that at least two people in the class can swim.

Statement B: No

There is nothing to suggest that Molly and Jeremy must be among those in the class who can ride a bike.

Statement C: No

As we do not know how many people there are in the class or how many people exactly can ride a bike, it is not possible to draw this conclusion.

Statement D: No

There is nothing to suggest that there is an association between Molly and Jeremy's abilities.

Statement E: No

As mentioned in statement A, we can establish that there are at least four people in the class. If there were more than four people in the class, this statement would be true. However, if we consider a situation with four people in the class, there would be an equal number of people who can swim and those who cannot.

Logical Puzzles

Logical puzzles are common, and can be divided into single parameter, multiple parameter and visual puzzles. Single parameter puzzles tend to be relatively straight forward, and can often be answered without drawing diagrams. Multiple parameter puzzles however often require you to use your laminated booklet whilst visual puzzles can sometimes incorporate an element of spatial reasoning.

Let's look at a practice question. Take 60 seconds to answer *Example Question 4*. Make a note of your answer before moving on to the explanation.

Example Question 4

Tanya, Mairi, Belinda, Trevor and Trent went on holiday together. The weight of their luggage when they departed was 10, 13, 15, 18 and 22 kilograms (not in any order). During their holiday they went shopping together on numerous occasions. Everyone's luggage was heavier when they came home; 12, 20, 24, 26 and 28 kilograms (not in any order).

Trevor's luggage doubled in weight.

Mairi's luggage was the lightest when she came home.

On departure, Belinda's luggage was lighter than Tanya's and heavier than Trent's.

Trent's luggage was the heaviest when they can home.

How much did Trent's luggage weigh when he departed?

    A. 10 kilograms

    B. 13 kilograms

    C. 15 kilograms

    D. 18 kilograms

Single Parameter Puzzles

Single parameter puzzles are relatively straight forward as long as you read each of the rules carefully. In *Example Question 4* the only parameter present was the weight of the luggage. If you struggle to keep all of the facts in your head, simply write out the weights in a single line in your laminated notebook. Start by reading each rule in turn. Jot down the initial (or first two letters if multiple people have the same first initial) of the person to whom the weight corresponds to for each rule. By writing the initial above for the pre-holiday and initial below for the post-holiday weights you also save time.

This technique quickly allows you to visualise the rules even though they were presented as a text format, and quickly allows you to tackle single parameter questions with accuracy.

Example Question 4: Answer and Explanation

The correct option was C – 15 kilograms.

The first rule states that Trevor's luggage doubled in weight. The only possible combinations of departure weight and return weight are 10 kilograms increasing to 20 kilograms and 13 kilograms increasing to 26 kilograms.

Mairi's luggage was the lightest when she came home, and therefore her luggage must have weighed 12 kilograms when she returned. As everyone's luggage was heavier when they came home, her luggage must have weighed 10 kilograms on departure.

As a result, you can now conclude that Trevor's luggage must have increased from 13 to 26 kilograms.

On departure, Belinda's luggage was lighter than Tanya's and heavier than Trent's. We know that Trevor and Mairi's luggage weighed 10 and 13 kilograms on departure respectively. Therefore, we can conclude that Trent, Belinda and Tanya's luggage weighed 15, 18 and 22 kilograms respectively on departure.

Top Tip: If you're struggling to retain each step, quickly draw it out in your laminated booklet.

Multiple Parameter Puzzles

Multiple parameter puzzles are more complicated, as they focus on multiple variables being present. As such, it's often more efficient to use your laminated booklet to visually represent the information as you're working your way through the question.

Let's look at a practice question. Take 60 seconds to answer *Example Question 5*. Make a note of your answer before moving on to the explanation.

Example Question 5

Brian, Arun, Chang and Charlie are each in charge of different school societies and were given the choices of visiting a zoo, museum, art gallery or architectural centre for their school society trip. The group sizes for the societies were 10, 18, 29 and 34 (not in any particular order).

The number of students in Arun and Chang's group put together is less than the number of students in Charlie's group.

Brian went on the trip with the largest group of students.

29 students went to the art gallery.

The museum does not accept a group size greater than 15.

Which of the following statements must be true?

    A. Charlie went to the zoo.

    B. Brian went to the architectural centre or the zoo.

    C. Arun went to the museum.

    D. There were 18 students in Chang's group.

Solving Multiple Parameter Puzzles

The easiest way to approach multiple parameter questions is to:

1. Create a grid in your laminated booklet.

2. Read each rule in turn, linking relevant items in your grid.

3. Look out for any logical inferences which can be made as a result.

4. Analyse each statement in turn, selecting the correct option.

In *Example Question 5* there are three parameters: name, destination and group size. Each of the parameters has four variables. To create a grid you will therefore need three columns (for the parameters) and four rows (for the variables). The order in which you place each item in the respective columns is irrelevant, simply list all variables for each column in a new row.

Once this is completed, you can then analyse each rule in turn. Draw a line connecting each variable based on the rule, but don't forget to also connect any logical inferences you can make as a result. Once you've connected everything you can, you're in a position to analyse each of the answer statements one by one, identifying the correct response.

Example Question 5: Answer and Explanation

Creating a grid and applying the rules gives us:

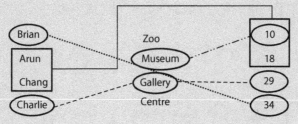

We know that Brian went on the trip with the largest number of students. We can therefore link Brian to 34.

We are told that the combined number of Arun and Chang's group is less than the number of students in Charlie's group. The only combination of numbers that is possible for this statement to hold true is 10 and 18, which in total are less than both 29 and 34. As we already know that Brian went with the largest group, we can now deduce that Charlie must have gone with the group of 29. We know that 29 students went to the art gallery, and so now know this was Charlie's group.

The museum does not accept a group size greater than 15 and so the size of the group visiting the museum must have been 10.

We can now analyse each statement in turn:

A. Charlie went to the zoo

This is incorrect as we know that Charlie went to the art gallery.

B. Brian went to the architectural centre or the zoo

This is correct. We know that Brian was in a group of 34, and that the museum must have taken the group of 10. As we also know that Charlie went to the art gallery, this leaves the zoo and architectural centre as options.

C. Arun went to the museum

All we know is that Arun and Chang were in the groups of 10 and 18 students, of which one went to the museum. We cannot however deduce which of Arun and Chang went to the museum.

D. There were 18 students in Chang's group

We only know that Chang was in a group of 10 or 18 students but we cannot say which.

Let's look at a practice question. Take 60 seconds to answer *Example Question 6*. Make a note of your answer before moving on to the explanation.

Example Question 6

$$\bigstar = \heartsuit + \Uparrow$$

$$\Uparrow + \Diamond = \heartsuit + \heartsuit$$

$$\heartsuit = \Diamond + \Diamond$$

$$\Uparrow + \Uparrow = \heartsuit + \heartsuit + \ ?$$

Which shape will make the last equation true?

A. Diamond

B. Heart

C. Arrow

D. Star

Approaching Visual Puzzles

There are numerous different ways in which visual puzzles can present. Some will involve spatial relationships between items or people, such as the order in which they might be sitting at a table or in the cinema, whilst others will combine logic and symbols.

Example Question 6: Answer and Explanation

We can solve the question by creating equations:

1. ♡ = 2 ◇
   ◇ = 0.5 ♡

2. ⇧ + ◇ = 2 ♡
   ⇧ + 0.5 ♡ = 2 ♡
   ⇧ = 1.5 ♡

3. 2 ⇧ = 3 ♡
   Missing symbol = ♡

The fundamental approach to visual puzzles is the same as for written ones, but the visual element can easily throw candidates. When dealing with spatial relationships between items or people it is often easiest to quickly draw this out in your laminated booklet. For symbol questions, try to convert them into equations. Doing this will allow you to solve the questions quickly and easily.

Statistical and Figural Reasoning

Having a solid grasp of maths, in particular basic probability and Venn diagrams, will certainly help you approach this part of the Decision Making section.

Let's look at some practice questions. Take 2 minutes to answer *Example Questions 7 and 8*. Make a note of your answers before moving on to the explanations.

Example Question 7

42 students are asked whether they like bananas, strawberries or apples.

20 students like bananas. 16 students like strawberries. 16 students like apples. 10 students like strawberries and bananas, and 4 of these students like apples as well.

Which of the following diagrams represents this?

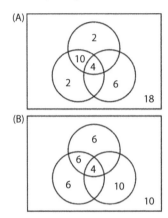

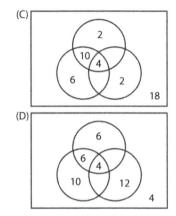

Example Question 8

Timothy is having a birthday party and would like to either go to the ballpark or trampolining. His parents gave the rest of his school class a survey about what their ideal birthday party would be to help them decide. They were given a choice of ice skating, rollerblading, going to the ballpark, trampolining and going to the waterpark.

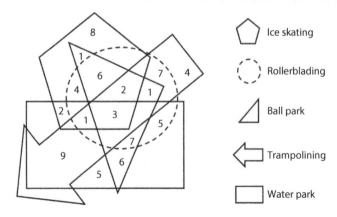

Based on the diagram, how many children in the class chose going to the ballpark as one of their activities?

    A. 23

    B. 24

    C. 26

    D. 27

Approaching Venn Diagrams

Venn diagrams allow you to visualise all of the possible logical relationships between different sets of information. For Decision Making, it's important you understand the basics of Venn diagrams (Example Question 7), as well as how to interpret more abstract versions (Example Question 8).

Example Question 7: Answer and Explanation

This was an example of a more traditional Venn diagram. You were presented with some data and had to pick the correct Venn diagram which displayed this data.

When filling in Venn diagrams, always start in the centre – in this case, the number of students who like all three fruits. By focusing on the statement that '10 students like strawberries and bananas, and 4 of these students like apples as well', we can deduce that there will be 4 students in the area where all three circles overlap and 6 students in the area where two circles overlap. Hence, we can eliminate options A and C. From this we can also identify that the bottom right circle represents students who like apples. As we know that 16 students like apples in total, option B can be eliminated leaving option D as the correct answer.

There are two ways in which you can approach these types of question. Either you use the elimination technique, such as outlined earlier, whereby each time you analyse a piece of information, you eliminate potential answers until left with just one. Alternatively, sometimes it's easier to draw a Venn diagram in your laminated booklet based on the information first, then pick the answer option which matches.

Top Tip: When filling in a Venn diagram don't forget to subtract the values already accounted for!

Example Question 8: Answer and Explanation

This was a slightly more abstract representation of a similar concept. These are common in the exam, and require you to correctly identify the overlap area. But be careful – don't forget to read the question carefully, as there may be more to it!

The number of children can be worked out by counting all the numbers present within the triangle, which represents those who chose going to the ball park. This shows 26 children in the class chose the ballpark. But the question stem says that Timothy wants to go to the ballpark, and his parents gave 'the rest' of his class the survey. As such you need to add Timothy to the results, giving 27 children in the class in total.

Let's look at a practice question. Take 1 minute to answer *Example Question 9*. Make a note of your answer before moving on to the explanation.

Example Question 9

In a fitness class, there is a warm up of 14 press-ups. Anyone unable to do 14 or more receives a punishment. Jessica can do 10 press-ups without ever failing, however, the chance of her successfully doing each subsequent press-up halves.

What is the probability of her receiving a punishment?

   A. 1 in 8

   B. 1 in 1024

   C. 15 in 16

   D. 1023 in 1024

Probabilistic Reasoning

Having a strong grasp of basic probability will certainly help, although you do not need any knowledge beyond that of GCSE level.

When calculating probabilities, the probability that a certain outcome, A, will happen is given by the formula:

$$P(A) = \frac{\text{Total number of ways A could occur}}{\text{Total number of possible outcomes}}$$

- If an outcome is *certain* to happen, it has a probability of 1.
- If an outcome is *impossible*, it has a probability of 0.

Let's use the formula to look at some basic examples involving a dice:

- What is the probability I roll a six?

$$P(A) = \frac{\text{Total number of ways A could occur}}{\text{Total number of possible outcomes}} = \frac{1}{6}$$

In this case, there is only one way to achieve the outcome, but we have six possible outcomes in total.

- What is the probability I roll a one *or* a six?

$$P(A) = \frac{\text{Total number of ways A could occur}}{\text{Total number of possible outcomes}} = \frac{2}{6} = \frac{1}{3}$$

This time we have two possible ways A could occur: rolling a one or a six. As such, the odds of getting a one *or* a six is a third.

- What is the probability I roll a one *then* a six?

This introduces the concept of conditional probabilities, where one event is dependent on another – in this case, the odds of rolling a six after having already rolled a one. To calculate conditional probabilities, we need to multiply the odds of each event happening together. We have already calculated the odds of rolling a one as 1 in 6, and of rolling a six as 1 in 6. As such, the odds of rolling a one then a six will be:

$$\frac{1}{6} \times \frac{1}{6} = \frac{1}{36}$$

Top Tip: Conditional probability questions often involve an item being removed after the first step, such as a coloured ball from a bag. If this is the case, don't forget to reduce the total number of items left when starting step 2 of your calculation.

Example Question 9: Answer and Explanation

We can now apply the earlier to solve *Example Question 8*. We can ignore the first 10 press-ups since the chance of them being successful is 1, and multiplying by 1 has no effect.

We can start by calculating the probability of Jessica successfully completing the 4 subsequent press-ups:

$$\frac{1}{2} \times \frac{1}{4} \times \frac{1}{8} \times \frac{1}{16} = \frac{1}{1024}$$

But remember this is the chances of her being successful – so the probability of getting a punishment is:

$$1 - \frac{1}{1024} = \frac{1023}{1024}$$

Top Tips for Decision Making

- Use your pen and laminated answer booklet.
- Draw diagrams to visualise the information.
- Learn basic probability.
- Practice all the different question formats.
- Section 1 BMAT questions can help!
- Keep an eye on the time – you only have 64 seconds per question.

Time for some practice! Try answering the following *29 questions*. You have 32 minutes to answer all questions. Detailed explanations are provided. Good luck!

Questions

Question 1

Several businesses including Factories, Heli and NXM are in the same industrial area. Their buildings are either black or white and are represented by symbols in the aerial view of the area in the following.

Factory X42 is closer to NXM than Factory P38

When people leave Heli via the street B exit, Factory K1 is visible to the left

Factory R2D is a white factory

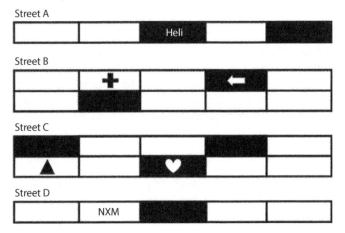

Which factory is represented by the cross?

    A. Factory X42

    B. Factory P38

    C. Factory K1

    D. Factory R2D

Question 2

I have 60 beans in a jar. I remove a quarter of the beans and sort them into white and black. I discard the white ones and then put the black ones back, along with an equal number of red beans.

Given the proportion of white beans in the jar and the sample I removed was 1/3, what is the ratio of white beans to black beans now?

    A. 5:8

    B. 2:5

    C. 2:3

    D. 3:8

Question 3

Some fluffballs are thupps. All snargles are fluffballs. No fluffballs are groshters. Some snargles are lulas. Some groshters are thupps.

Which of these statements are definitely true?

    A. Some lulas are fluffballs.

    B. No snargles are thupps.

    C. Some thupps are both groshters and snargles.

    D. All fluffballs are groshters.

Question 4

Three train companies have trains running between Manchester and Edinburgh. Company A is known for their budget train tickets as they offer the cheapest rates every day except Mondays and Fridays. Company B offers to beat the prices of other companies if a customer provides them with a quote for the cheapest ticket on offer. Company C has decided to drop the prices of their Saturday tickets further which makes it the cheapest rate.

Place 'Yes' if the conclusion does follow. Place 'No' if the conclusion does not follow.

    A. If considering train travel on a Saturday from Manchester to Edinburgh, it is best to travel with Company A (Yes/No).

    B. David wants to travel from Edinburgh to Manchester on Tuesday. If he would like the cheapest ticket, he should approach Company B with a quote from Company A (Yes/No).

    C. Company B sells the cheapest tickets (Yes/No).

    D. If travelling to Manchester to Edinburgh on a Saturday and returning to Manchester on the following day, it is best to book both tickets with Company C (Yes/No).

    E. There is no benefit in approaching Company B with a ticket quote from Company A for travel on a Friday (Yes/No).

Question 5

Should train companies reduce the cost of annual season tickets for commuters?

Select the strongest argument from the following statements:

    A. Yes, as some commuters have complained about high costs previously.

    B. Yes, more commuters are using other means of transport such as cycling and buses.

    C. No, commuters earn enough money to pay for annual season tickets.

    D. No, the revenue from season tickets is needed to carry out essential engineering works.

Question 6

Drug M and drug N are both used for a certain illness.

About 300 out of 3,000 people who took drug M are cured. Of the people who took drug N, 10% of people were cured.

About 20% of people taking drug M relapsed after 2 years and 25 out of 75 people taking drug N reported a relapse after 2 years.

Considering *only* the chance of cure and relapse, is drug M a better choice?

    A. No, the likelihood of cure is 10% for drug N compared to 1% for drug M.

    B. No, the chance of cure and relapse are the same for both drugs.

    C. Yes, the chance of cure is higher with drug M.

    D. Yes, the risk of relapse is lower with drug M.

Question 7

Harvey is selling items from his house at a car boot sale. The numbers represent the number of items.

The hexagon represents items that are brand new.

The diamond represents items that cost more than £20.

The triangle represents electronic items.

The oval represents his sister's belongings.

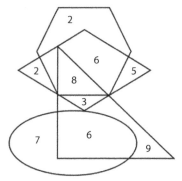

Which of the following statements is true?

    A. All of his sister's belongings are electronic items.

    B. The number of brand new items costing more than £20 was exactly four-fold greater than the number of brand new items costing less than £20.

    C. More than half of the electronic items cost less than £20.

    D. Some of the brand new items belonged to his sister.

Question 8

There are eight people queuing up to be seen by the casualty nurse. Mr A is more than three positions behind Mr B. Miss C was not the first to report at reception. Mrs D, Mr E and Mr F are all in odd numbered positions, and Mr G is three positions ahead of Mr H. Mr H is in the back half of the queue, standing in between Mrs D and Mr E.

Which of the following MUST be true?

    A. Mr A is last in the queue.

    B. Mr F is 5th in the queue.

    C. Mr H is second to last in the queue.

    D. Mr G is 1st in the queue.

Question 9

Should Heathrow airport in London build a third, new runway?

Select the strongest argument from the following statements:

    A. Yes, as this would make Heathrow comparable in size with other large European airports.

    B. Yes, as the local economy would benefit.

    C. No, another runway would mean more flights that would produce more carbon dioxide and therefore cause environmental damage.

    D. No, flights would cause noise pollution for the surrounding residential areas.

Question 10

Children were asked to request sandwich fillings for their school picnic. They were given a choice of ham, cheese, egg, lettuce, pickle and mayonnaise.

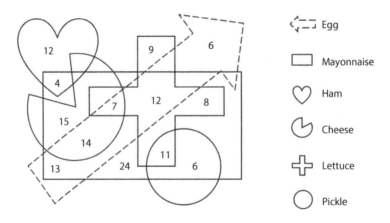

Based on the diagram, how many students had sandwiches with egg, mayonnaise and cheese, but no lettuce?

A. 12

B. 13

C. 14

D. 15

Question 11

Luke has an un-biased dice. The probability that it will land on the number 5 is 1 in 6.

He throws the dice 6 times and the dice lands on 6 every time.

Luke decides that the probability cannot be 1 in 6.

Is he correct?

A. Yes, because he threw the dice 6 times and it did not land on 5.

B. Yes, because the outcome of the first 6 throws suggests that the probability that the dice lands on 6 is greatest.

C. No, because the outcome of previous throws has no effect on the probability that it will land on 5.

D. No, he would need the outcome of more throws for this statement to become true.

Question 12

Various chefs were showcasing their skills at the London cooking show. Of these chefs, none were men working in the pastry industry.

Place 'Yes' if the conclusion does follow. Place 'No' if the conclusion does not follow.

A. The chefs at the London cooking show who work in the pastry industry were women (Yes/No).

B. There were more female chefs than male chefs at the London cooking show (Yes/No).

C. There were no male chefs at the London cooking show (Yes/No).

D. Of the female chefs at the London cooking show, the majority work in the pastry industry (Yes/No).

E. No chefs at the London cooking show work in the pastry industry (Yes/No).

Question 13

Luke, Lyla, Hans, Chu and Daria are members of an athletics club. They are doing timed 100 metres sprints as part of the selection for the regional championships.

Chu is faster than Lyla.

Hans is slower than Daria.

Luke is faster than Hans but slower than Lyla.

Which of the following must be true?

    A. Luke is faster than Daria.

    B. The fourth fastest runner was Daria.

    C. The slowest runner is Hans.

    D. The fourth fastest runner was Luke.

Question 14

Anita's grandmother, Edith, gave birth to Elisa when she 25 years old. Elisa was 28 years old when Anita was born.

Frederick, Anita's father, and Elisa married in 1984. Saskia is Anita's older sister.

Which of the following statements must be true?

    A. Anita was born in 1984, Saskia in 1990, Elisa in 1956.

    B. Anita was born in 1992, Saskia in 1994, Elisa in 1970.

    C. Anita was born in 1987, Saskia in 1985, Elisa in 1959.

    D. Anita was born in 1990, Saskia in 1988, Elisa in 1947.

Question 15

A scientist is testing the effect of two antibiotics, antibiotic A and antibiotic B, on bacteria X and bacteria Y. She grows the bacteria in a Petri dish with different antibiotics and at different temperatures. The number of bacteria is then counted in colony forming units (CFU).

Temperature (°C)	Antibiotic	Number of bacteria X counted (CFU)	Number of bacteria X and bacteria Y counted (CFU)
40	None	3,000	5,200
40	A	200	2,000
50	B	3,000	4,400
60	B	3,000	4,700
60	A+B	2,700	4,600

Which of the following statements *cannot* be concluded from the information provided in the chart?

    A. Antibiotic A is more effective against bacteria X than bacteria Y.

    B. The growth of bacteria Y is inhibited to a greater degree by antibiotic B than antibiotic A.

    C. Antibiotic B works best at 50°C.

    D. Antibiotic B reduces the antibacterial effects of antibiotic A against bacteria X.

Question 16

Students have applied for a science scholarship programme. Those who are studying at least three science subjects are being interviewed first.

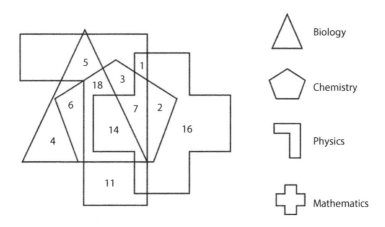

How many students are interviewed in the first round?

    A. 27

    B. 39

    C. 42

    D. 49

Question 17

Seven friends are at the cinema to watch a movie. They all sit in one row. Ronnie always sits in the middle. Wayne is sitting in one of the spaces on Ronnie's right-hand side. Mark is sitting in between Wayne and Jack. Wayne is not allowed to sit next to Ronnie. James is last on the left from Ronnie. George and Tim are also watching the movie with their friends.

Which of the following statements must be true?

    A. George is sitting next to James.

    B. There are three people sat between George and Mark.

    C. Wayne is sitting the furthest away from James.

    D. Tim is sitting between George and Ronnie.

Question 18

Students in a class were asked where they had been on holiday over the last 2 years:

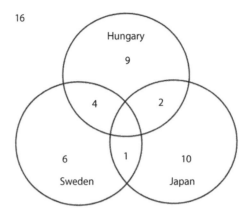

Which one of the following statements is true?

A. There are 32 students in the class.

B. More students have been on holiday to Japan compared to the number of students who have been to Hungary.

C. Sweden is the least visited country by the students out of the three countries over the last 2 years.

D. Every student has been to at least Hungary, Sweden or Japan over the last 2 years.

Question 19

Kyle, Celene, Tariq and Maria went shopping together to buy shoes. They each bought different coloured shoes which included the colours red, green, blue and white (not in any order). The cost of the shoes was £20, £22, £40 and £60 (not in any order).

Kyle's shoes were exactly twice as expensive as Maria's shoes. The most expensive pair of shoes was white. Tariq's shoes were cheaper than Kyle's.

Who bought white shoes?

A. Kyle

B. Celene

C. Tariq

D. Maria

Question 20

On Mr Jones' farm, there are 40 sheep and 30 chickens. Two thirds of the chickens are brown. The rest of the chickens are white. Half the sheep are brown. None of the sheep are black.

Place 'Yes' if the conclusion does follow. Place 'No' if the conclusion does not follow.

A. There are 20 white sheep (Yes/No).

B. There are more brown chickens than there are sheep (Yes/No).

C. There are no white sheep (Yes/No).

D. There are the same number of brown goats and brown sheep (Yes/No).

E. There no black chickens or black sheep on Mr Jones' farm (Yes/No).

Question 21

There are two gambling machine games in an arcade:

LuckyCoins:
- 40 p to play.
- 50 coins of different colours of which 10 are white.
- 3 coins are randomly selected and if 2 or more are white you win £1.

NameANumber:
- £1.5 to play.
- Press a number from 0 to 9 inclusive.
- If the number pressed is the same as the randomly generated number of the machine you win £4.

You have £10 and can only use one of the machines. Which game gives you the highest amount of money at the end, if you use as much of the £10 as possible?

A. LuckyCoins

B. NameANumber

C. No difference between the games

D. Not possible to tell

Question 22

Nancy and Edward are playing table tennis with each other.

The probability that Edward will lose a table tennis match is 0.8.

If Nancy and Edward play three matches in total, the likelihood that Edward will win exactly two matches is greater than the chance of him winning all three matches.

Is this correct?

A. No, because the chance of Edward winning all three matches is 0.08 and 0.032 for winning exactly two matches.

B. No, because there is a 0.2 chance of winning in both situations.

C. Yes, because the chance of Edward winning exactly two matches is 0.0032 and 0.08 for all three matches.

D. Yes, because the probability of Edward winning exactly two matches is 0.096 and 0.008 for all three matches.

Question 23

A group of friends go on a Ferris wheel and they each sit in a carriage on their own.

Jamie's carriage is directly opposite the closed carriage.

Farah and Felix are also directly opposite each other.

Alan is on carriage 4.

Ai is on a carriage that is between Farah and the closed carriage.

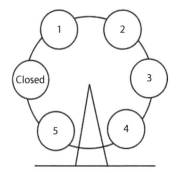

Who is sitting in carriage 2?

    A. Farah

    B. Ai

    C. Felix

    D. Jamie

Question 24

A group of friends are eating dinner at a restaurant.

Four of them ate bread before eating a three-course meal. Two of them ate a main and a desert. Four people ate a starter and a main dish. Those who ate two courses did not eat any bread. One person ate bread and one main dish.

Which of the following best represents this?

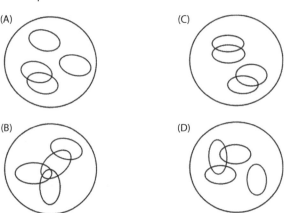

Question 25

A mobile phone company is analysing two of their products.

The chance that mobile X90 breaks is one in ten and two in forty for mobile X360.

Mobile X90 requires charging twice every 2 days.

Mobile X360 needs to be charged three times every 72 hours.

Considering *only* the chance of breaking and frequency of charging, is mobile X90 the better product?

    A. Yes, because the mobile X90 has a lower frequency of charging.

    B. Yes, because the mobile X90 has a smaller chance of breaking.

    C. No, because both mobiles have the same chance of breaking and the same frequency of charging.

    D. No, because both mobiles have the same frequency of charging, but mobile X90 has a higher chance of breaking.

Question 26

The charts compare the difference in the disease prevalence for two continents over a 100-year period. Disease numbers are represented where 1 = 1 million people.

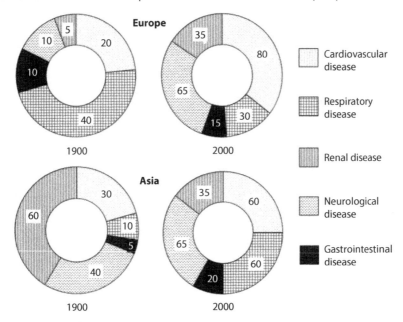

Which of the following statements can be concluded from these charts?

    A. More Europeans are affected by neurological diseases and respiratory diseases in 2000 compared to 1900.

    B. The biggest increase across both continents over the 100-year period is cardiovascular disease.

C. Fewer Asians are affected by renal disease and cardiovascular disease in 2000 compared to 1900.

D. In both 1900 and 2000, gastrointestinal disease has always been the least prevalent disease type in both Europe and Asia.

Question 27

It is the school baking competition. Mel, Paul, Tamal, Sue, Mary and Nadia are competing in the final round. The judges have placed their bakes in order from first to sixth place on a table, with the winner closest to the trophy at one end of the table.

Three bakes have been placed between Paul and Sue's.

Mel came first in the final round.

Paul is further from the trophy than Nadia.

There are three bakes between the trophy and Mary.

Tamal's bake was closer to Sue's than Paul's.

Who was in third place in the final round?

A. Nadia

B. Mary

C. Tamal

D. Sue

Question 28

Should the UK government continue to fund the building of nuclear weapons?

Select the strongest arguments from the following statements:

A. Yes, continual financing of nuclear weapons has so far acted as a deterrent for global nuclear war.

B. Yes, the existence of nuclear weapons makes other countries scared and intimidated of the UK.

C. No, the UK has spent billions of pounds on nuclear weapons up until now.

D. No, the UK should not spend on unnecessary things when there is so much debt on which the money could be better spent.

Question 29

The government sets time-targets of 4 hours per patient for all UK casualty departments. The intended aim is that at least 95% of patients will be seen and treated within 4 hours of their arrival.

Welford Hospital and Tarth Hospital have their casualty departments' time-target published for a 10-year period.

Year	% of casualty patients seen within 4 hours	
	Welford	Tarth
2005	89.5	86.1
2006	87.7	94.4
2007	86.1	99.5
2008	98.1	98.3
2009	93.4	98.2
2010	95.3	96.8
2011	88.5	90.6
2012	90.9	98.2
2013	85.5	87.9
2014	89.4	86.8
2015	87.2	94.5

Which of the following statements is true?

A. Welford casualty department in 2010 has seen and treated a lower proportion of patients compared to Tarth.

B. Tarth casualty department in 2008 saw more patients within the 4-hour target than Welford.

C. Tarth casualty department has passed the 4-hour target for twice as many years as Welford has.

D. Tarth's best performing year for seeing and treating casualty patients within 4 hours was also Welford's worst performing year.

Answers

Question 1 – B

Factory X42 is closer to NXM than Factory P38, which means that the triangle or heart or cross may be Factory X42 and the arrow or cross may be Factory P38.

The arrow must be Factory K1 as it is visible on the left when people leave Heli via street B. Therefore, Factory P38 must be the cross.

For completeness sake, we know that R2D is a white factor and so it must be represented by the triangle. Therefore, Factory X42 is represented by the heart.

Question 2 – D

A quarter of 60 means removing 15 beans. Of these, 5 will be white and are discarded.

To begin with, the number of white beans is 60/3 = 20. There are now 15 white beans since 5 were discarded. The number of black beans remains at 40.

Therefore, the ratio is 15:40, which is 3:8.

Question 3 – A

The Venn diagram shows the information we know, where the '?' shows areas that may or may not intersect.

A.   Is definitely true since some snargles are lulas and all snargles are fluffballs, then all the lulas that are snargles are also fluffballs.

B.   May or may not be true since although we know that some thupps are fluffballs, they may not intersect with the subgroup of snargles.

C.   Although some thupps are groshters and some thupps are snargles, no thupp is both a groshter and a snargle, since all snargles are fluffballs and no fluffballs are groshters.

D.   As per C.

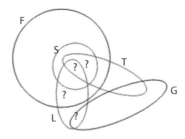

Question 4 – No/Yes/No/No/Yes

A.   No

Company C provides the cheapest rate on a Saturday and therefore it would be best to travel with Company C, not Company A.

B. Yes

Company A provides the cheapest rates on a Tuesday. Company B will beat the price if provided with a quote for the cheapest ticket on offer. Therefore, this conclusion does follow.

C. No

Company B will offer to beat the ticket prices of other companies and therefore have the scope to sell the cheapest ticket, but this only applies to situations where a customer provides them with the quote for the cheapest ticket on offer.

D. No

Company C will sell the cheapest ticket on a Saturday but this is not the case for travel on a Sunday, where Company A or Company B (if given a quote from Company A) will offer a cheaper ticket.

E. Yes

Although Company A sells the cheapest tickets on most days of the week, it does not on Fridays. Company B will only beat the prices of other companies if they are provided with a quote for the cheapest ticket on offer. Therefore, it is true that there would be no benefit in approaching Company B with a quote from Company A.

Question 5 – D

A is not the strongest argument as it refers only to 'some commuters'.

B could be viewed as irrelevant to the question or that it attempts to imply that commuters are using other means of transportation due to the cost of annual season tickets.

C is based on the assumption that commuters 'earn enough money'.

D is the strongest argument as it is relevant to the question being asked and gives a solid reason by bridging the need for revenue from season tickets with 'essential engineering works'.

Question 6 – D

The chance of cure with drug M is 300 out of 3,000, which can be simplified to 1 in 10. One in 10 is equal to a 10% chance. The chance of cure with drug N is 10%.

Therefore, both drugs have the same chance of cure.

There is a 20% chance of relapse with drug M and this is equal to a 1 in 5 chance. Twenty five out of 75 people taking drug N relapsed, which equates to a 1 in 3 chance.

Therefore, the risk of relapse lower with drug M.

Question 7 – C

Statement A is not true as there are 7 items represented by an area of the oval shape which does not overlap with the triangle representing electronic items.

Statement B is incorrect. The number of brand new items costing less than £20 is represented by areas where the hexagon does not overlap with the diamond. There are 2 items in this area. The number of brand new items costing more than £20 is represented by the area where the diamond and hexagon overlap. There are 8 electronic items and 6 other items, giving a total of 14 items which is seven-fold greater.

Statement C is true. The total number of electronic items can be calculated by adding all the numbers within the triangle, which equates to 26 items. Those that cost less than £20 are represented by the areas which do not overlap with the diamond. By adding the 6 items that belong to his sister and the 9 items that do not, we can see that 15 items, that is more than half of the electronic items, cost less than £20.

Statement D is incorrect as the oval representing his sister's belongings and the hexagon representing brand new items do not overlap.

Question 8 – A

Mrs D, Mr E and Mr F are all in an odd-numbered position, so they are in either position 1, 3, 5 or 7. If Mr H is in the back half of the queue between Mrs D and Mr E, then Mrs D and Mr E occupy positions 5 and 7 (in no particular order). That means, that as Mr H is standing between Mrs D and Mr E, Mr H is in position 6. Mr G is three spaces ahead in position 3. As all the odd numbered positions apart from position 1 are taken, Mr F must be in position 1.

Mr A must be more than three spaces behind Mr B, so we know Mr A is behind Mr B. Whether Mr B is in position 2 or position 4, as Mr A must be more than 3 spaces behind Mr B. Therefore, Mr A must be last in the queue.

Position	Person
1	F
2	B/C
3	G
4	B/C
5	D/E
6	H
7	D/E
8	A

Question 9 – C

A. What positive benefit does making Heathrow in similar size to another airport have for people? This weaker argument can be strengthened by giving a reason as to why a larger airport is beneficial: for example, to the local economy or for international businesses.

B. This argument could be much stronger if reasons were given as to why the local economy would benefit – that is increased employment and potential for local businesses to expand. Instead, a blanket statement that cannot be justified does not make for a strong argument.

C. A logical and reasoned argument for not having a further runway and the negative impact it can have. There are reasons given which support the conclusion.

D. This is a weaker argument, as the airport by definition will already have flights going in and out, causing noise. A more robust argument would be to show that *more* flights, as a result of an additional runway, would cause *more* noise pollution.

Question 10 – C

The area where the arrow, rectangle and partial circle, which represent egg, mayonnaise and cheese respectively, overlap should be identified. The area which overlaps with the cross, which represents lettuce, should then be eliminated. Therefore, there are 14 students who had the sandwiches with this combination.

Question 11 – C

The key to this question is that as the dice is un-biased, the probability that the dice lands on 5 will always be 1 in 6 regardless of the outcome of previous throws.

Question 12 – Yes/No/No/No/No

A. Yes

We know from the passage that there were no male chefs at the London cooking show working in the pastry industry. Therefore, any chefs who work in the pastry industry and were present at the cooking show must have been women.

B. No

The passage does not give any information with regards to the numbers of proportion of male and female chefs.

C. No

There were no male chefs who worked in the pastry industry at the cooking show but this does not mean that were no male chefs at the cooking show.

D. No

As established in statement A, if there were any chefs at the cooking show who work in the pasty industry, they must be women. However, this does not imply that the majority of female chefs work in the pastry industry.

E. No

The passage states that there are no male chefs working in the pastry industry at the cooking show, but there is still scope for there to be female chefs who work in the pastry industry at the show.

Question 13 – C

If we write out each statement it would be as follows:

- Chu > Lyla
- Hans < Daria
- Hans < Luke < Lyla

If these statements are then placed in order, the order would be:

- Hans < Luke < Lyla < Chu

We know that Daria is faster than Hans but we do not know whether he is faster than Luke, Lyla or Chu. Therefore, statement C is the only statement that must be true.

Question 14 – C

The key to this question is to look at the age differences and to note that as Edith is not mentioned in any of the answer options, we do not need to consider the information provided about her.

The age difference between Elisa and Anita is 28 years. Statement A and statement C are the only ones that fulfil this.

Saskia is Anita's older sister and therefore must have been born before Anita. Statement C is therefore the correct answer.

Question 15 – D

A can be concluded: There are 3,000 CFU of bacteria X when no antibiotics are used and there are 200 CFU when antibiotic A is used. Therefore, antibiotic A reduces the number of bacteria X by 2,800 CFU. There are 5,200 CFU of bacteria X and Y when no antibiotics are used and as there are 3,000 CFU of bacteria X, we can deduce that there are 2,200 CFU of bacteria Y. There are 2,000 CFU of bacteria X and Y when antibiotic A is used and as there are 200 CFU of bacteria X, we can deduce that there are 1,800 CFU of bacteria Y. Therefore, antibiotic A reduces bacteria Y by 400 CFU.

B can be concluded: By considering that there are 3,000 CFU of bacteria X at both temperatures, we can deduce that there are 1,400 CFU of bacteria Y at 50°C and 1,700 CFU at 60°C. We have already established that without antibiotics there are 2,200 CFU of bacteria Y. Therefore, antibiotic B reduces bacteria Y by 800 CFU and 500 CFY at 50°C and 60°C respectively. We know from the previous statement that antibiotic A reduces bacteria Y by 400 CFU.

C can be concluded: We have established in statement B that bacteria Y is reduced by 800 CFU at 50°C and 500 CFU at 60°C. The effect on bacteria X is not significant as it is clear that antibiotic B has no effect on bacteria X at both temperatures.

D cannot be concluded: We know that at 60 degrees, antibiotic B does not have any effect on bacteria X. Therefore the 300 CFU reduction in bacteria X is due to antibiotic A. The reduction on bacteria X by antibiotic A at 40°C is 2,800 CFU. Therefore at 60 degrees, where both antibiotic A and antibiotic B are used, there is indeed a reduction in the antibacterial effects against bacteria X. However, it is not possible to tell whether this is due to antibiotic B being used also or the increase in temperature.

Question 16 – B

The first step is to identify the areas where three or more shapes overlap. This allows us to identify 18 students studying Biology, Physics and Chemistry, 7 student studying Physics, Mathematics and Chemistry and 14 students studying Mathematics, Biology and Chemistry. Therefore 39 students must have been interviewed in the first round.

Question 17 – C

Following is a pictorial representation of the information provided. The crucial part to recognise is that we cannot tell which specific seats George and Tim are sitting in.

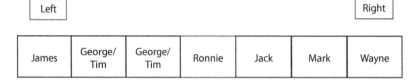

Left						Right
James	George/ Tim	George/ Tim	Ronnie	Jack	Mark	Wayne

Question 18 – C

Statement A is incorrect: The total number of students is calculated by adding all of the numbers seen in the diagram, which equates to 48 students. It is important not to forget to include the 16 students who have not been to Hungary, Sweden or Japan.

Statement B is incorrect: In total, there are 13 students who have been to Japan and 15 students who have been to Hungary.

Statement C is true: 11 students have visited Sweden, compared to the 15 students who have visited Hungary and 13 students who have visited Japan.

Statement D is incorrect: There are 16 students who have not been to Hungary, Sweden or Japan, as indicated by the number in the Venn diagram that is not within any of the circles.

Question 19 – B

Kyle's shoes were exactly twice as expensive as Maria's shoes. We can therefore allocate £40 to Kyle and £20 to Maria.

Tariq's shoes were cheaper than Kyle's, so they must be £22.

This leaves Celene, whose shoes must have cost £60. As the most expensive pair of shoes were white, we can now deduce that Celene bought white shoes.

Question 20 – No/No/No/No/Yes

A. No

   The passage tells us that there are 20 brown sheep and no black sheep. However, there is no further information provided that allows us to deduce what colour the other 20 sheep are.

B. No

   As two thirds of the chickens are brown and there are 30 chickens, there must be 20 brown chickens. As half the sheep are brown and there are 40 sheep, there must be 20 brown sheep.

C. No

   The passage tells us that half the sheep are brown and none of the sheep are black, but this does not allow us to deduce whether or not there are white sheep.

D. No

   There are indeed the same number of brown chickens and brown sheep, but this statement refers to brown goats, which are not mentioned in the passage.

E. Yes

   We know that the chickens are either brown or white and that there are no black sheep. Therefore, this statement logically follows.

Question 21 – B

LuckyCoins:

- The probability of getting a white coin (W) is 0.2.
- Therefore: W, W, ? $= 0.2^2 \times 1 = 0.04$.
- As there are 3 ways of getting this, $0.04 \times 3 = 0.12$.
- So probability of getting 2 or more white coins is 0.12.
- If there is a 0.12 chance of earning £1, then statistically you earn an average of £0.12 per go.

With 10 pounds, you could have 25 chances so would earn an average of £3.

Name a Number:

- The chance of getting the same number is 1 in 10.
- If there is a 0.1 chance of earning £4, then statistically you would earn £0.4 per go.

With £10, you could have 6 chances that would earn you an average of £2.4.

But, as you only used £9 so your total money (not winnings) at the end would be £3.40.

Question 22 – D

The probability that Edward will win a match is 0.2. There are three possible situations in which Edward will win exactly two matches:

P(WLW) or P(WWL) or P(LWW) $= 3 \times (0.2 \times 0.2 \times 0.8) = 0.096$

P(WWW) $= 0.2 \times 0.2 \times 0.2 = 0.008$

Question 23 – A

By working through the information provided, we can allocate everyone to the following carriages:

A. Ai
B. Farah
C. Jamie
D. Alan
E. Felix

Question 24 – A

One separate circle represents those eating a three-course meal. The circle representing those who ate a main dish and a desert but no bread and the circle representing those who ate a starter and a main dish but no bread overlap. The overlapping area represents the fact that both groups of people ate a main dish and did not eat any bread. One separate circle represents those who ate bread and one main dish.

Question 25 – D

Both mobile X90 and mobile X360 require charging once every 24 hours.

The chance of mobile X90 breaking is 1 in 10. The chance of mobile X360 breaking is 2 in 40 which can be simplified to 1 in 20.

Therefore, mobile X90 has a higher chance of breaking.

Question 26 – B

Statement A is incorrect as the number of respiratory diseases fell in Europeans between 1900 and 2000.

Statement B can be concluded because in Europe, cardiovascular diseases increase 4-fold from 20 to 80 million, and in Asia from 30 to 60 million. This equates to an increase of 90 million cases, the largest of any of the diseases.

Statement C does not follow as although the number affected by renal diseases did fall, the number affected by cardiovascular diseases increased.

Statement D is incorrect as we can see that gastrointestinal diseases were not the least prevalent in 1900 in Europe.

Question 27 – C

If we work through each statement we can slowly identify the order of placement.

There are three bakes between Paul and Sue so it is best to write this out as:

Paul/___/___/___/Sue

Mel came 1st, we have been told that the winner's bake is closest to the trophy at one end of the table.

Trophy/Mel/Paul or Sue/___/___/___/Paul or Sue

Paul is further from the trophy than Nadia so it is impossible for him to have come 2nd. Therefore, we now know that Sue and Paul must have come 2nd and 6th respectively. There are three bakes between the trophy and Mary so she must have come 4th.

Trophy/Mel/Sue/___/Mary/___/Paul

For Tamal's bake to be closer to Sue's than Paul's, he must have come 3rd. We now know that Nadia must have come 5th, which fulfils the statement that Paul is further from the trophy than Nadia.

The final order is therefore:

Trophy/Mel/Sue/Tamal/Mary/Nadia/Paul

Question 28 – A

A is the only argument that addresses the point of continual funding. Financing of nuclear weapons in the past and its positive outcome has been used to argue support for the conclusion.

B is a weaker argument as we are not questioning the existence of nuclear weapons as a whole.

C is a weaker argument as this is just a statement that a lot of money has been spent in the past.

For D, no explanation has been given as to why funding the building of nuclear weapons is unnecessary, just that it is an opinion.

Question 29 – C

Tarth casualty department had at least 95% of patients seen and treated within 4 hours in 2007, 2008, 2009, 2010 and 2012 (5 years). Whereas Welford only had more than at least 95% seen and treated within 4 hours in 2008 and 2010.

A. The key piece of information that is missing 'within 4 hours'. We cannot tell if Welford has seen a fewer proportion of patients.

B. We do not know the absolute population of either hospital so we cannot come to this conclusion.

D. Tarth's best performing year was 2007 (99.7% patients seen within 4 hours) whereas Welford's worst performing year was 2013 (85.5% patients seen within 4 hours).

CHAPTER 3

Quantitative Reasoning

Overview

The Quantitative Reasoning (QR) Section is one the most time pressured parts of the UKCAT examination. It challenges students to solve mathematical problems by applying logic and reasoning. Students who aren't studying maths beyond GCSE often feel disadvantaged in this Section. But the truth is: they aren't! As the UKCAT website says, the QR Section *'assumes familiarity with numbers to the standard of a good pass at GCSE. However items are less to do with numerical facility and more to do with problem solving'*. In other words, the emphasis is on logic and reasoning, not complex calculations.

Format of the Section

Students will be presented with 9 Scenarios. Each of these Scenarios contains 4 associated questions. This gives a total of 36 questions. Each question has 5 answer options. You have 25 minutes in which to complete all 36 questions (including 1 minute of reading time).

Each Scenario begins with a short passage of introductory text. This is followed by some data. The data can be presented in a number of ways, including:

- Tables
- Charts/pie charts
- Graphs
- 2- and 3-dimensional shapes
- Diagrams
- Pure text with no pictorial representation

Sometimes the answer options include 'Can't Tell'. This means that it is *not possible* to calculate the answer to the question, based on the available information. It does not mean that after performing calculations, you disagree with the other answer options. If you think that it is possible to work it out, but you have arrived at a different answer, then you may have made a mistake.

Mathematical Knowledge

The level of mathematical knowledge required is quite basic. You need to be familiar with:

- Basic arithmetic
- Fractions, decimals and ratios
- Averages
- Percentages
- Common formulas
- Geometrical formulas

The key challenges include: correctly identifying which data to use, applying logic and reasoning to solve problems, and doing it all under immense time pressure. Even the most basic question can become complicated when you add in the dreaded time factor!

One interesting application of basic arithmetic is drug calculations. These have become more common in the application process, also featuring in many medical school MMI interviews. In reality, all the information required can usually be found within the question stem, but the unfamiliarity with the concept can easily throw candidates.

Strategy

This section feels – and is – very time pressured. So it is imperative that you become less reliant on using a calculator by performing mental arithmetic.

You have an average of 40 seconds per question. But some questions will take far longer to answer. Strategy, therefore, becomes essential. You need to 'gain time' on easy questions, so that you can spend more on the challenging ones.

Whenever looking at a question, you should ask yourself three things:

1. Do I need to do any calculations?
2. Do the numbers work?
3. Can I eliminate any answer options?

Many questions in QR require no calculations at all. They simply involve correctly reading data from the information presented. It seems straightforward, but working under time pressure can make it very challenging in practice.

Students preparing for the QR section often believe they will need to use a calculator for every question. This couldn't be further from the truth. The numbers in QR often tend to work quite nicely. They may look complex at first, but are often designed in such a way that they can be calculated in your head, or quickly using the booklet provided. There are, of course, questions where you will need to use your calculator.

Top Tip: When revising, give yourself 6 'tokens' for the QR section. Each time you use a calculator during a full set of 36 QR questions, it means you've used 1 token. This simple rule will help you think twice before using your calculator in the future. Eventually, this will make you faster!

You are not allowed to bring a pocket calculator into the exam. You have to use the on-screen one. You can activate this by clicking the 'calculator' button in the top left corner of the screen or clicking alt + c. The on-screen calculator is very basic, effectively limiting you to: addition, subtraction, multiplication and division. There is also a square root button. But that's it! Again, this highlights the fundamental principle of QR that it has less to do with numbers, and more to do with problem solving.

Top Tip: Using the on-screen calculator is significantly more time consuming than using a pocket calculator. So, when revising from a textbook, always use your computer's basic calculator (e.g. in the Windows start bar) to answer questions. This allows you to replicate the UKCAT's on-screen calculator – with all the associated difficulties.

Every question in QR has five possible answers. It is, however, often possible to eliminate one or more answer options straight away. Some will use the wrong units; others will be in the wrong order of magnitude. So, even if you are tempted to guess on a question, always try to eliminate some implausible options first.

The 'flag' function is particularly important in the QR because of the intense time pressure. Some questions are more time consuming than others. If you're not vigilant, you may find yourself struggling to finish the section. When you encounter a particularly time-consuming question, your best option is to select a sensible answer (having eliminated obviously incorrect options), before 'flagging' it and moving quickly on.

Remember: Every question is worth 1 mark. So, you're better off finishing the section and answering all the easy 1 mark questions than you are answering fewer difficult questions and running out of time. The best 'game strategy', rather than the cleverest answers, will ultimately lead to success.

Common Themes

In the Quantitative Reasoning Section there are many common themes along with subtle tricks to catch you out. The following Example Question Sets will demonstrate how these work in practice. By the end of this section, you will feel much better prepared to tackle the QR section of the UKCAT.

Refer to the following *Example Set 1*. Keep in mind the three golden rules as you work your way through:

1. Do I need to do any calculations?

2. Do the numbers work?

3. Can I eliminate any answers?

Set a timer for 160 seconds and make a note of your answers before moving on to the explanations.

Example Set 1

Using the table of conversions between metric units and imperial units, answer the following questions:

Metric Unit	Imperial Unit
5 kilometres	3 miles
8,000 metres²	2 acres
9 litres	2 gallons
13 kilometres²	5 miles²

1. A car drives 126 miles in 98 minutes. It then stops at a service station for 24 minutes. It then resumes its journey, covering 72 more miles in 58 minutes. What was its average speed in kilometres per hour?

   A. 110 miles per hour

   B. 66 kilometres per hour

   C. 110 kilometres per hour

   D. 66 miles per hour

   E. 126.9 kilometres per hour

2. A car has a miles-per-gallon rate of 30. If the same car travels 225 kilometres, how many litres of fuel can it expect to consume?

   A. 56.25

   B. 33.75

   C. 20.25

   D. 4.5

   E. 1

3. An area of woodland covers 2.5 miles² in total. How many acres does it cover?

    A.   1,625

    B.   812.5

    C.   240.4

    D.   16.25

    E.   6.5

4. There is a flood that covers 9 acres of land with water that is, on average, 2.5 metres deep. If there are 1,000 litres in a cubic metre of water, how many gallons of water are there on the flooded land?

    A.   20

    B. 8×10^6

    C. 8×10^7

    D. 2×10^7

    E. 20×10^7

Example Set 1: Answers and Explanations

Question 1

ANSWER: C – 110 kilometres per hour

The average speed for a journey is equal to *total* distance covered divided by the *total* journey time (which includes periods when the car wasn't moving).

First determine the total distance covered, which is 126 + 72 = 198 miles.

In kilometres, this is (198/3) × 5 = 330 kilometres.

Then determine the total journey time, which is 98 + 24 + 58 = 180 minutes or 180/60 = 3 hours.

So, overall, the car's average speed was 330/3 = 110 kilometres per hour.

Question 2

ANSWER: C – 20.25

First determine its kilometre per-gallon rate: (30/3) × 5 = 50 kilometres per gallon.

So, to travel 225 kilometres, the car would have to consume 225/50 = 4.5 gallons of fuel.

This is equal to (4.5/2) × 9 = 20.25 litres of fuel.

Question 3

ANSWER: A - 1,625

First determine this area in kilometres²: 2.5/5 × 13 = 6.5 kilometres².

There are 1,000 × 1,000 = 1,000,000 meter² to a kilometres², so the area of the wood land covers 6,500,000 metres².

This area in acres is therefore (6,500,000/8,000) × 2 = 1,625 acres.

Question 4

ANSWER: D - 2 × 10⁷

9 acres of land is the same as (9/2) × 8,000 = 36,000 metres².

If the water is 2.5 metres deep, we are dealing with a volume of water that is 36,000 × 2.5 = 90,000 metres³.

This is the same as 90,000 × 1,000 = 90,000,000 litres, which is equal to (90,000,000/9) × 2 = 20,000,000 gallons or 2 × 10⁷ gallons.

This question was quite tricky with multiple steps and calculations to perform. It's a true test of your ability to perform basic arithmetic under time pressure! In addition, it utilises a favourite formula of the UKCAT:

$$\text{Speed} = \frac{\text{Distance}}{\text{Time}}$$

This is a commonly used formula and one you must be familiar with and quickly be able to rearrange in the exam.

Now is a good time to revise similar shapes. Take a look at the two shapes in the following, Shapes A and B:

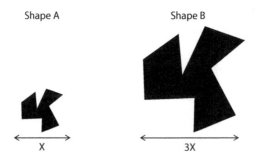

Shape A

Shape B

X

3X

How many times larger is the area of Shape B compared to Shape A? If they were 3-dimensional, how many times larger would the volume of Shape B be?

Remember that with similar shapes, they have a constant difference in size in all dimensions to each other. As such, Shape B has an area $3^2 = 9$ times larger than Shape A, and a volume of $3^3 = 27$ times larger.

For the next questions, please refer to *Example Set 2*. Allow yourself 160 seconds to complete the next four questions, making note of your answers before moving on to the explanations.

Example Set 2

An ecologist is examining how the climate affects the growth of a particular species of moss. She looks at a sample of rocks on which the moss is growing and records the average percentage coverage of the rocks' surface area by moss. She displays this data on the following graph, along with rainfall data for the surrounding area (rainfall is expressed in millimetres).

Average rainfall and percentage coverage are displayed on a bi-monthly basis, that is, for each variable. The x-axis labels show the average figure for the month shown and the following month. So 'Jan'. shows the average rainfall and percentage across both January and February. The first dataset on the graph shows percentage coverage and rainfall at the beginning of 2017 and subsequent datasets are displayed chronologically, left to right.

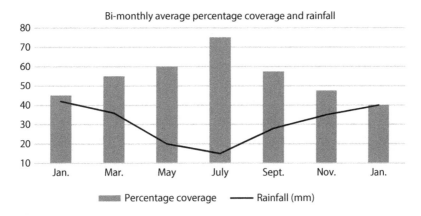

1. What was the average percentage coverage in the November to December period?

   A. 58%

   B. 57.5%

   C. 49%

   D. 47.5%

   E. 35%

2. What was the percentage decrease in average rainfall between the May–June period and the July–August period?

   A. 33.3%

   B. 25%

   C. 50%

   D. 28.6%

   E. 30%

3. What was the relative change in percentage coverage between the periods of May–June and July–August?

   A.   25%

   B.   15%

   C.   20%

   D.   30%

   E.   20.83%

4. What was the average monthly percentage coverage in 2017, rounded to the nearest percent?

   A.   32%

   B.   27%

   C.   57%

   D.   28%

   E.   63%

Example Set 2: Answers and Explanations

Question 1

ANSWER: D – 47.5%

Reading directly from the chart shows that average percentage coverage in the November–December period was 47.5%. Find the 'Nov'. value on the x-axis (since each month labelled on the axis also includes data for the following month) and read across to the y-axis. This is an example of where you simply need to read the data from the chart without performing any calculations.

Question 2

ANSWER: B – 25%

In the May–June period, average rainfall was 20 millimetres. In the July–August period, average rainfall was 15 millimetres. Therefore, there was a decrease in average rainfall of 5 millimetres between these two periods.

So the percentage decrease was (5/20) × 100% = 25%.

Question 3

ANSWER: A – 25%

Looking at the chart, we see that in May–June average percentage coverage was 60% and in July–August this figure rose to 75%. Therefore, the change in percentage coverage is 75% – 60% = 15%. Note that this is the *absolute* change in percentage coverage.

The question asks for the *relative* change in percentage coverage, in other words, the change in percentage coverage relative to the original value.

So if coverage was initially 60%, the relative change is (15/60)% × 100% = 25%.

Question 4

ANSWER: D – 28%

From the introduction, we know that the first dataset was in 2017. Hence the first bar shows average percentage cover in January–February 2017. We can then add up the figures shown by the bars for the whole year, which gives:

$$45 + 55 + 60 + 75 + 57.5 + 47.5 = 340$$

Note we do not include the data in the last bar because that gives data from the beginning of 2018.

As the question asks for the average *monthly* percentage coverage, and because we have worked the 'total' for the year, we have to divide this figure by 12, which is 28.333% or 28% to the nearest percent.

Percentages

Percentage based questions are common in the UKCAT. The two formulae you must know are:

$$\text{Calculating a percentage: } \frac{\text{Given amount}}{\text{Total amount}} \times 100$$

$$\text{Calculating the percentage change: } \frac{\text{Difference}}{\text{Original}} \times 100$$

Top Tip: A common mistake made under exam pressure when calculating the percentage change is to divide by the final value instead of the original. Be careful and pay attention!

To help you avoid using the calculator unnecessarily in the exam, it's helpful to learn some of the common percentage conversions. Whilst you will undoubtedly know most of these, learning some of the trickier ones will help you quickly spot tricks and shortcuts you can use by converting into fractions to save time.

- $1/2 = 0.5 = 50\%$
- $1/3 = 0.33 = 33.33\%$
- $1/4 = 0.25 = 25\%$
- $1/5 = 0.2 = 20\%$
- $1/6 = 0.167 = 16.7\%$
- $1/7 = 0.143 = 14.3\%$
- $1/8 = 0.125 = 12.5\%$
- $1/9 = 0.11 = 11.11\%$
- $1/10 = 0.1 = 10\%$

For the next questions, refer to *Example Set 3*. Allow yourself 160 seconds to complete the next four questions, making note of your answers before moving on to the explanations.

Example Set 3

Roger has gone to the supermarket to buy a ready-made lasagne. The price of Antonio's Amazing Lasagne is £5.35 per packet whilst the Budget Lasagne is £4.00. He looks at the nutritional information of the two different packages:

Antonio's Amazing Lasagne

	Per 100 grams	Per Quarter Pack
Calories (kilocalories)	152	190
Fat (grams)	7.4	9.25
- of which saturated fat (grams)	3.6	4.5
Sugar (grams)	4.0	5.0
Salt (grams)	0.6	0.75

Budget Lasagne

	Per 100 grams	Per Half Pack
Calories (kilocalories)	200	600
Fat (grams)	9.8	29.4
- of which saturated fat (grams)	6.6	19.8
Sugar (grams)	5.7	17.1
Salt (grams)	0.8	2.4

1. What is the weight of one packet of Antonio's Amazing Lasagne?

   A.   125 grams

   B.   400 grams

   C.   500 grams

   D.   600 grams

   E.   Can't Tell

2. What percentage of the Budget Lasagne is made of fat?

   A.   6%

   B.   6.5%

   C.   10%

   D.   16.5%

   E.   Can't Tell

3. The Budget Lasagne weights 600 grams per pack. Roger has invited 4 friends for dinner and everyone will eat 300 grams of lasagne. How much will it cost him if he buys them all Budget Lasagne?

   A.   £7.00

   B.   £8.00

   C.   £10.00

   D.   £12.00

   E.   £15.00

4. It transpires that there was a labelling error for the Budget Lasagne, and the calorie count was in fact 20% higher than labelled. How many calories are there per pack of Budget lasagne?

   A.   720 kilocalories

   B.   1,200 kilocalories

   C.   1,320 kilocalories

   D.   1,440 kilocalories

   E.   2,880 kilocalories

Example Set 3: Answers and Explanations

Question 1

ANSWER: C – 500 grams

On the surface, this question looks like it's not possible to answer. But you have been presented with values, both per 100 grams and per quarter pack. You can therefore calculate the ratio between them. If you look at the sugar content of Antonio's Amazing Lasagne, you don't need a calculator to see that the 'per quarter' value is 125% of the 100 grams value. Therefore, there are 1.25 multiples of 100 grams in a quarter pack. So, a quarter pack must weigh 125 grams. A full pack weighs 4 times a quarter pack, so 500 grams.

Question 2

ANSWER: C – 10%

This is an incredibly simple question to answer. Yet many struggle. You do not need to perform any calculations as you have been presented with a percentage table in your data. You have all the values per 100 grams. Anything per 100 is effectively synonymous with percentages. So, all you have to do is read off the value – which is 9.8%. Sometimes numbers are rounded slightly up or down. If this is the case, you will almost certainly be presented with 'Can't Tell' as an answer option. But remember: 'Can't Tell' means it's *not possible* to calculate the answer; not that you disagree with the other options.

Question 3

ANSWER: D – £12.00

As Roger is having 4 friends over for dinner, there will be 5 people eating in total: the four friends plus Roger himself. As each person eats 300 grams of lasagne, he will need to buy 1,500 grams. The Budget Lasagne comes in packets of 600 grams. So, he will need to buy 3 packets (1,800 grams), since he cannot buy half a packet. Therefore, the price is $3 \times £4.00 = £12.00$.

Question 4

ANSWER: D – 1,440 kilocalories

The original table told you that there were 600 kilocalories per half pack. With the labelling error, this means that there was in fact 720 kilocalories per half pack. For a full pack, you need to double this value, giving you 1,440 kilocalories.

Top Tip: When faced with recipe questions, remember that if you 'buy' something you must round up to the nearest whole integer, as you can-not buy fractions of items. However, if you 'use' an ingredient, you can work in fractions.

Ratios and Proportions

This question introduced the concept of ratios and proportions. But what's the difference?

A ratio is when we compare one component to another, whilst a proportion is comparing one component to the total.

For example, let's say we wanted to bake a cake using one part butter and two parts flour. As such, the ratio of butter to flour is 1:2, whilst the proportion of butter is 1/3.

For the next questions, refer to *Example Set 4*. Allow yourself 160 seconds to complete the next four questions, making note of your answers before moving on to the explanations.

Example Set 4

A language school teaches classes in seven languages. Each pupil at the school only studies a single language. The proportion of pupils learning each language at the beginning of the academic year is shown in the following pie chart.

Number of pupils doing each language course

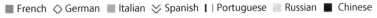

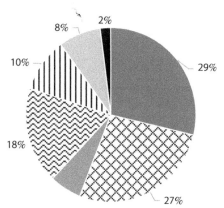

1. If 20 students are studying Russian, how many students are studying Italian?

   A. 27

   B. 20

   C. 35

   D. 15

   E. Can't Tell

2. Assume the total number of pupils is 150. Twelve new students join to study Portuguese. What is the new percentage of people studying Spanish to the nearest whole number?

   A.   17

   B.   26

   C.   28

   D.   29

   E.   16.67

3. Assume that the number of people in the school is 500. If the number of students studying Chinese doubles and the number of students studying German increase by a fifth, what is the percentage increase in pupils at the school?

   A.   2

   B.   5.4

   C.   11.4

   D.   37

   E.   7.4

4. The school decides to introduce a new language, Arabic part-way through the year. Twenty new students start the Arabic course. Assuming that 6 students studied Chinese at the beginning of the year, what is the mean number of students per subject after the introduction of Arabic?

   A.   77.5

   B.   40

   C.   37.5

   D.   45.7

   E.   38

Example Set 4: Answers and Explanations

Question 1

ANSWER: D – 15

If 8% are studying Russian, then 1% of the group is 20/8 = 2.5. Adding up the rest of the percentages leaves 6% for Italian (100 – (27 + 29 + 2 + 8 + 10 + 18) = 6).

Therefore 6 × 2.5 = 15 students study Italian.

Question 2

ANSWER: A – 17

The number of people studying Spanish is $0.18 \times 150 = 27$. An increase of 12 brings the total to 162.

As the number of people studying Spanish has stayed the same, the new percentage is $27/162 \times 100\% = 16.67\%$ or 17% to the nearest whole number.

Question 3

ANSWER: E – 7.4

The number of students studying Chinese is $0.02 \times 500 = 10$. If this doubles, there is an increase of 10 Chinese students. The number of students studying German is $0.27 \times 500 = 135$. An increase of a fifth is 27.

Therefore the total number of new pupils is $10 + 27 = 37$. This represents a percentage increase of $37/500 \times 100\% = 7.4\%$.

Question 4

ANSWER: B – 40

If 6 students are studying Chinese at the beginning of the year and 2% of students study Chinese at this point, then overall there are $(6/2) \times 100 = 300$ students.

Arabic students increase the number of total students to 320. Therefore, the average number of students per subject after the introduction of Arabic is $320/8 = 40$.

For the next questions, refer to *Example Set 5*. Allow yourself 160 seconds to complete the next four questions, making note of your answers before moving on to the explanations.

Example Set 5

My garden is represented in the following diagram. It has a peculiar shape, one that faintly resembles an 'S'. It has a central rectangular area and, adjoining this, there are two identical regions at each end of the garden. These regions are made up of a smaller rectangle and a triangle. The length of each smaller rectangle is half the length of the larger rectangle.

I also have a roller, which may be represented as a cylinder of circumference 200 centimetres and length of 75 centimetres.

Not to Scale

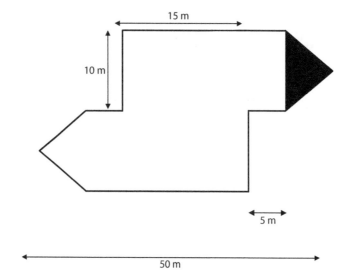

1. What is the area of the region shaded black in centimetres squared?

   A.   1,250,000

   B.   750,000

   C.   625,000

   D.   125

   E.   62.5

2. The central rectangle consists of a lawn, whereas the adjoining areas are covered by patio. How many rotations of the roller are required to flatten the lawn?

   A.   2

   B.   100

   C.   200

   D.   350

   E.   300

3. I am thinking of downgrading to a new house with a garden two-thirds the size of this one. What would be the surface area of my new garden?

   A.   412.5 metres²

   B.   275 metres²

   C.   525 metres²

D. 350 metres²

E. 433.33 metres²

4. I might sell off some of the land on the adjoining areas so that the triangular areas are lost. If I decided to put up a fence around my modified garden, what would be the cost of this in pounds if materials cost £6.50 per metre of fencing needed?

A. 585

B. 520

C. 487.50

D. 455

E. 90

Example Set 5: Answers and Explanations

Question 1

ANSWER: C – 625,000

The length of the triangles *together* can be gained from $50 - 15 - (2 \times 5) = 25$ metres.

Therefore the length (or 'height') of one triangle is $25/2 = 12.5$ metres.

The area of one triangle is given by ½ base × height $= (10/2) \times 12.5 = 62.5$ metres².

Note the question asks for the answer in centimetres², so this answer needs to be multiplied by 100^2 which gives a final answer of $62.5 \times 10,000 = 625,000$ centimetres².

Question 2

ANSWER: C – 200

The surface area of a roller (at least, on the surface in contact with the ground) is $200 \times 75 = 15,000$ centimetres². This is equal to $15,000/10,000 = 1.5$ metres².

 This flattened out would give…

The lawn is $15 \times 20 = 300$ metres² in surface area.

Therefore, as one full rotation of the roller will cover 1.5 metres² of lawn, to flatten the lawn will require $300/1.5 = 200$ rotations.

Question 3

ANSWER: D – 350 metres²

The central rectangle has an area of 15 × 20 = 300 metres².

A single adjoining section has an area of the smaller rectangle (5 × 10 = 50 metres²) and the triangle (12.5 × (10/2) = 62.5 metres²) which is 112.5 metres². As there are two of them, this gives a total adjoining surface area of 2 × 112.5 = 225 metres².

The total area of the garden at the moment is 300 + 225 = 525 metres².

The new garden would have a surface area of (2 × 525)/3 = 350 metres².

Question 4

ANSWER: A – 585

The length of the perimeter of the modified garden would be

$$(2 \times 15) + (4 \times 10) + (4 \times 5) = 90 \text{ metres}$$

Therefore, the cost of fencing would be 90 × 6.50 = £585.

Geometry

A sound grasp of basic geometry is essential for the UKCAT. You're expected to be able to calculate the perimeter and area of basic 2-dimensional shapes, and the surface area and volume of basic 3-dimensional shapes.

2-Dimensional Shapes		
Shape	Perimeter	Area
Square	4 S	S^2
Rectangle	(2 × L) + (2 × H)	L × H
Parallelogram	S1 + S2 + S3 + S4	B × H
Circle	$2\pi r$ or πd	πr^2
Triangle	A + B + C	½ × B × H
3-Dimensional Shapes		
Shape	Surface Area	Volume
Box	2lw + 2lh + 2wh	l × w × h
Sphere	$4\pi r^2$	$4/3\ \pi r^3$
Cylinder	$2\pi r(r + h)$	$\pi r^2 h$

Although knowledge to 'the standard of a good pass at GCSE' requires you to know that $\pi = 3.14$, it is very rare that QR questions require you to work with π as an absolute number. You do get questions relating to circles and – more rarely – spheres and cylinders. But, in these cases, the questions will either state '$\pi = 3$', making it easier to work with, or be designed in such a way that they express π as part of the answer – not as an absolute number.

> **Top Tip:** When faced with complex abstract shapes, such as in Example Set 5, always try to simplify the shape by breaking it into its constituent parts.

Summary of Quantitative Reasoning

Remember: The Quantitative Reasoning section of the UKCAT is less to do with math and more to do with logical reasoning. This cannot be emphasised enough! The on-screen calculator is cumbersome and awkward to use, not to mention time consuming. So avoid it if you can. Practice your mental arithmetic regularly to build both accuracy and confidence.

There are a few formulae that come up frequently, and which you should know well:

$$\text{Speed} = \frac{\text{Distance}}{\text{Time}}$$

$$\text{Percentage} = \frac{\text{Given amount}}{\text{Total amount}} \times 100$$

$$\text{Percentage change} = \frac{\text{Difference}}{\text{Original}} \times 100$$

$$\text{Average} = \frac{\text{Sum of numbers}}{\text{Number of numbers}}$$

Time for some practice! Try answering the following *9 Practice Sets*. You have 24 minutes to answer all questions. Detailed explanations are provided. Good luck!

Questions

Scenario 1

Two friends, Matthew and John, have decided to race each other on bikes around the woods. They have set up three checkpoints: A, B and C. They both start at point A, with Matthew cycling from A to B to C then back to A. John, however is cycling from A to C to B to A. The distance from A to B is 4 miles and from B to C is 6 miles. It takes Matthew 20 minutes to cycle from A to B. He completes the entire course in 90 minutes. Matthew arrives back at point A half an hour before John.

Question 1

How much faster did Matthew cycle compared to John?

    A.   25%

    B.   One third

    C.   4/9

    D.   0.75

    E.   Can't Tell

Question 2

Assuming Matthew cycles at a constant speed throughout, how far is it between points C and A?

    A.   4 miles

    B.   6 miles

    C.   8 miles

    D.   10 miles

    E.   18 miles

Question 3

After the race, it transpired that John had gotten lost between points C and B, increasing his race distance. In total John cycled 22 miles. What was his average speed?

    A.   11 miles per hour

    B.   12 miles per hour

    C.   13 miles per hour

    D.   14 miles per hour

    E.   15 miles per hour

Question 4

The friends decide that as cycling is very good for keeping fit, by burning approximately 500 kilocalories per hour, they should do 2 hours a week for all but 4 weeks in the year. How many calories per year will they each burn as a result?

A. 24,000 calories

B. 26,000 calories

C. 48,000 calories

D. 52,000 calories

E. 48,000,000 calories

QR Scenario 2

James is currently driving to and from his office every Monday to Friday but feels it's time to upgrade to a new car. He is undecided about which car to get so he has created the following table:

	Audi A4	Audi A5	Mercedes C Class
Price	£23,600	£28,670	£24,450
Engine size	2.0 litres	1.8 litres	1.8 litres
0–60 miles per hour	9.2 seconds	7.6 seconds	8.7 seconds
Horsepower	134 BHP	167 BHP	153 BHP
Top speed	134 miles per hour	143 miles per hour	140 miles per hour

Question 1

If James wishes to upgrade the sound system on the Audi A5, he needs to pay an additional £716.75. What is the percentage increase in total price?

A. 2%

B. 2.25%

C. 2.5%

D. 2.75%

E. 3%

Question 2

To buy the Audi A4, James takes out a loan. The terms of the loan require him to pay a 25% deposit followed by 24 monthly payments of £800. How much extra will James have to pay the aforementioned list price?

A. £1,400

B. £1,475

C. £1,500

D. £1,625

E. £2767.50

Question 3

The Mercedes C Class has a fuel tank size of 67.5 litres and a fuel economy of 40 miles per gallon. One gallon is approximately 4.5 litres. How far can the Mercedes C Class travel on a third of a tank of petrol?

A. 182.25 miles

B. 200 miles

C. 300 miles

D. 400 miles

E. 600 miles

Question 4

James commutes 25 miles to work every day. If he bought the Audi A4, his fuel efficiency would be 10 miles per litre of petrol. Currently, petrol costs £1.40 per litre. How much would it cost him to commute to and from work every week?

A. £17.50

B. £26.25

C. £35.00

D. £49.00

E. Can't Tell

Scenario 3

Noradrenaline is a drug used in critical care units to increase the blood pressure of sick patients in shock. It has to be given as a continuous infusion, the strength of which varies as standard strength (4 milligrams of Noradrenaline diluted in 50 millilitres of saline), double strength (8 milligrams of Noradrenaline diluted in 50 millilitres saline) and quadruple strength (16 milligrams Noradrenaline diluted in 50 millilitres saline).

Question 1

A patient is receiving an infusion of standard strength Noradrenaline at a rate of 0.5 micrograms per kilogram of body weight per minute. He weighs 70 kilograms. How much Noradrenaline is he receiving per hour?

A. 21 micrograms

B. 35 micrograms

C. 2.1 milligrams

D. 35 milligrams

E. 2.1 grams

Question 2

A 60 year old gentleman weighing 62.5 kilograms is requiring 3 milligrams Noradrenaline per hour. How many syringes of double strength Noradrenaline will he require per 24 hours?

A. 3

B. 5

C. 6

D. 9

E. 18

Question 3

Noradrenaline is sold in vials containing 4 micrograms of powder each, costing £11.55 per vial. Saline costs £0.10 per 10 millilitres container. To draw up the solution, staff require a 50 millilitres syringe (costing £0.45) and a needle (costing £0.12). What is the cost of drawing up a quadruple strength Noradrenaline infusion?

A. £12.22

B. £12.62

C. £24.17

D. £46.87

E. £47.27

Question 4

The average cost per night for a patient staying in an intensive care unit is £1,500. The intensive care unit at a district general hospital has eight beds, and runs at an average occupancy of 75% throughout the year. What is the annual cost of patients staying in the intensive care unit?

A. £2,190,000

B. £3,285,000

C. £3,832,500

D. £4,380,000

E. Can't Tell

Scenario 4

The following graph shows the average rates of water flow at various points along a river in both summer and winter for this year.

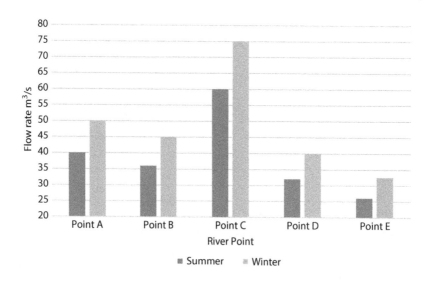

Question 1

What was the average flow rate along the whole river in the summer?

    A. 48.5 m³/s

    B. 38.4 m³/s

    C. 39.4 m³/s

    D. 38.8 m³/s

    E. 37.4 m³/s

Question 2

Last year, the average flow-rate at Point B in winter was 40 m³/s. What has been the percentage change in flow-rate since then?

    A. 12.5% decrease

    B. 10% decrease

    C. 12.5% increase

    D. 5% decrease

    E. 11.11%

Question 3

A cubic metre of water weighs one metric tonne. How many tonnes of water flow past Point C in the summer over the course of a two- and three-quarter-hour period?

A. 594,000

B. 742,500

C. 9,900

D. 702,000

E. 594

Question 4

At another point, Point F, water flows at a rate of 30 m³/s in the summer. By examining trends on the graph, what can we estimate the flow rate in the winter to be?

A. 24 m³/s

B. 40 m³/s

C. 42 m³/s

D. 37.5 m³/s

E. Can't Tell

Scenario 5

White blood cells are produced to fight infections. There are five main types of white blood cell that collectively make up the total white blood cell count. These five cell types include: neutrophils, leucocytes, monocytes, eosinophils and basophils. The following is a table of blood results of three patients:

	Normal Values	Patient 1	Patient 2	Patient 3
Haemoglobin (g/dL)	13–17	10.4	13.8	14.3
White Cell Count (×10⁹/L)				
Total	3–10	15.8	22.5	13.3
Neutrophils	2–7.5	8.9	15.3	11.2
Leucocytes	1.5–4	5.3	2.7	1.5
Platelets (×10⁹/L)	150–400	155	440	330

Question 1

What proportion of the white blood cells are made up by cells other than neutrophils and leucocytes in Patient 2?

    A. 1/3

    B. 1/4

    C. 1/5

    D. 1/6

    E. Can't Tell

Question 2

When they repeated the blood tests the next day, the platelet count of Patient 3 had decreased by 20%. What was his platelet count the next day?

    A. 124

    B. 264

    C. 297

    D. 332

    E. 396

Question 3

The estimated blood volume of patient 1 is 6 litres. How many grams of haemoglobin does his blood contain?

    A. 624 grams

    B. 1,040 grams

    C. 3,120 grams

    D. 6,240 grams

    E. 8,280 grams

Question 4

Patient 2 is treated with the antibiotic Meropenem, costing £10 per half gram. He requires 0.5 grams of Meropenem, three times per day for 7 days. This 7-day course costs six times as much as a standard 5-day course of the antibiotic Erythromycin. How much does a standard 5-day course of Erythromycin cost per day?

    A. £5.00

    B. £7.00

C. £14.00

D. £35.00

E. £70.00

Scenario 6

Mike and Sarah are buying a house together. On the ground floor there are two receptions rooms (3 × 6 metres) and (4 × 7 metres), a kitchen-diner (5 × 4 metres) and a hallway. The hallway is a quarter of the size of the largest reception room.

Question 1

What is the surface area of the ground floor?

    A. 66 metres^2

    B. 73 metres^2

    C. 77 metres^2

    D. 79 metres^2

    E. Can't Tell

Question 2

After buying the house, they build a semi-circular conservatory extension to the kitchen, increasing the overall area of the kitchen by 50%. To the nearest half metre, what is the diameter of the conservatory?

    A. 2.5 metres

    B. 3 metres

    C. 5 metres

    D. 6 metres

    E. Can't Tell

Question 3

Mike and Sarah bought their first house in 2016 for £225,000. It has subsequently increased in value by 6%. What is the value of their house today?

    A. £234,000

    B. £236,250

    C. £238,500

    D. £240,750

    E. £265,000

Question 4

Mike and Sarah's friends, Archie and Abbey, are looking to buy their first house and are offered a mortgage allowing them to borrow four times their deposit. Archie has been saving 15% of his £60,000 per year salary as a chartered accountant for the last 5 years. They have put down a deposit on a £340,000 house. Abbey has only been saving for 2 years but contributed 25% of her salary annually. How much does Abbey earn per year?

    A. £46,000

    B. £80,000

    C. £85,000

    D. £92,000

    E. £160,000

Scenario 7

A renowned design company is in the process of bringing out a new range of furniture. The furniture is to be made of moulded plastic.

The plastic has a density of 2 g/cm³. It costs £100 per metric tonne (1,000 kilograms).

When it arrives at the furniture factory, the plastic is in the form of small pellets which measure 3 centimetres in length. Their height is a third of their length, and their width is double their height. These pellets need to be melted down to be moulded.

The factory plans to produce chairs with odd-shaped legs. One chair leg can be regarded as a triangular prism, with a cross section shown in the following:

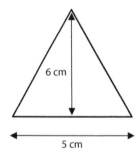

6 cm

5 cm

Question 1

The furniture factory has a processing vat which melts the plastic. The vat has a volume of 150 metres³. What number of pellets would fill half a vat?

    A. 12,500,000

    B. 25,000,000

    C. 1,250,000

    D. 2,500

    E. 1,250

Question 2

The chairs that the company are designing will have four legs. If each chair leg is 40 cm in length, what is the mass of plastic required to make the chair legs for a single chair?

A. 9.6 kilograms

B. 2.4 kilograms

C. 1.2 kilograms

D. 4.8 kilograms

E. 12 kilograms

Question 3

The plastic that is turned into chair legs is produced as long prisms with a triangular cross-section. These prisms are then cut into chair legs. If over the course of a single day the factory produces a prism that is 50 kilometres long in total, what would have been the cost of the plastic needed to produce it?

A. £150

B. £1,000

C. £7,500

D. £15,000

E. £150,000

Question 4

The factory also makes cabinets. However, the machine that makes cabinets is faulty, and 12.5% of the plastic that enters it is accidentally destroyed. If a cabinet *should* have a final weight 10.5 kilograms, what is the minimum number of pellets that are needed to ensure that one cabinet can be correctly made?

A. 7,000

B. 2,000

C. 1,000

D. 766

E. 1

Scenario 8

The Republic of Francissia has recently introduced a new tax system. Citizens have an income allowance before they have to pay income tax. After that, they pay tax as a percentage of their income over a given amount. At higher threshold levels of income there are higher rates of income tax. Certain members of society receive tax perks, for example, nurses only start paying income tax on earnings over FR$ 1,600. The tax system is summarised in the following table (the currency is the Francissian dollar, FR$):

Tax System in 2016	Tax System in 2017
Tax-free allowance up to FR$ 1,300	Tax-free allowance up to FR$ 1,400
20% on all income > FR$ 1,300 but ≤ FR$ 4,000	15% on all income > FR$ 1,400 but ≤ FR$ 3,800
30% on all income > FR$ 4,000 but ≤ FR$ 10,000	22% on all income > FR$ 3,800 but ≤ FR$ 10,000
40% on all income > FR$ 10,000	60% on all income > FR$ 10,000

Question 1

If a worker earned FR$ 1,300 in gross income 2016. What would their pay be after tax deductions if their wages in 2017 rose in line with an inflation figure of 1.5%, assuming they only pay income tax?

    A. FR$ 1,495

    B. FR$ 1480.75

    C. FR$ 1319.50

    D. FR$ 1316.58

    E. FR$ 1315.60

Question 2

What did a worker earning FR$ 12,250 receive in take-home pay in 2016, assuming income tax is the only deduction?

    A. FR$ 7,350

    B. FR$ 9,010

    C. FR$ 9,176

    D. FR$ 9,500

    E. FR$ 9,910

Question 3

What did a nurse earning FR$ 8,000 receive in take-home pay in 2017, assuming income tax is the only deduction?

A. FR$ 6,746

B. FR$ 6,716

C. FR$ 6,320

D. FR$ 6,260

E. FR$ 6,240

Question 4

If a person earned FR$ 5,000 in 2017 and 2016, what is the percentage reduction in the amount of tax paid in 2017 compared to 2016?

A. 216

B. 624

C. 5.19

D. 25.71

E. 34.62

Scenario 9

A zoo vet needs to sedate his elephants. To do this, he will use the special sedative *jumbodiaz-epane*. In elephants, the effective dose of *jumbodiazepane* is one microgram per kilogram of bodyweight (a microgram is one thousandth of a milligram), and the lethal dose is one and a half micrograms per kilogram of bodyweight.

An average male (bull) elephant weighs 3 tonnes (a tonne is 1,000 kilograms), a female weighs two-thirds of this, and a new-born calf weighs a quarter of its mother's weight.

An average zoo-vet weighs 80 kilograms.

Question 1

The vet has to sedate one bull elephant, two female elephants and three calves. What is the minimum weight of pure *jumbodiazepane* he needs to order?

A. 6,500 grams

B. 0.0078 grams

C. 0.0085 grams

D. 0.0065 grams

E. 8.5 grams

Question 2

The vet gives each elephant an injection of 10 millilitres. If he first prepares the sedation mixture in batches of one litre, how much pure *jumbodiazepane*, in grams, does he need to put into a batch to produce injections that will sedate elephants weighing one and a half tonnes?

    A. 150,000,000

    B. 150,000

    C. 1,500

    D. 150

    E. 0.15

Question 3

If the lethal dose of *jumbodiazepane* for a human is a tenth of a microgram per kilogram of body weight, how many zoo vets could be killed by the sedative by the amount needed to send to sleep a female elephant?

    A. 2.5

    B. 250

    C. 8

    D. 375

    E. 6.25

Question 4

Veterinary scientists have discovered that a compound found in peanuts lowers the tolerance thresholds of elephants to *jumbodiazepane* by one third. What is the largest weight of a pea-nut-eating elephant, in kilograms, that could be killed by 2.5 milligrams of *jumbodiazepane*?

    A. 5,000

    B. 2,500

    C. 2.5

    D. 5

    E. 3,750

Answers

Scenario 1

Question 1: B – one third

This is a simple question, but tests your knowledge of fractions and decimals, and your ability to quickly convert between them.

Matthew finishes the race in 90 minutes whilst John takes 120 minutes (you are told he finishes 30 minutes after Matthew). 120/90 = 1.333*.

Therefore Matthew cycles one third faster than John.

Question 2: C – 8 miles

This is a three-step calculation. You need to calculate:

1. Matthew's average speed: distance/time = 4 miles/20 minutes = 12 miles per hour.

2. Total distance travelled: You are told he cycles at a constant speed, and the total time spent is 90 minutes. Therefore, travelling at 12 miles per hour, he covers a total distance of 18 miles.

3. Subtract A to B and B to C from the total distance = 18 – 6 – 4 = 8 miles.

Question 3: A – 11 miles per hour

Remember the formula: speed = distance/time = 22/2 = 11 miles per hour.

Question 4: E – 48,000,000 calories

There are 52 weeks in a year, and they plan to cycle all but 4. Therefore they will cycle 48 times per year. On each occasion they plan to cycle for 2 hours, which gives a total of 96 hours per year. At 500 kilocalories per hour, this gives 48,000 kilocalories per year.

Remember your units:

Kilo × 1,000

Mega × 1,000,000

The answers are in calories, not kilocalories , therefore you have to convert 48,000 kilocalories to calories by multiplying by 1,000.

Scenario 2

Question 1: C – 2.5%

$$\text{The percentage change} = \frac{\text{Difference}}{\text{Original number}} \times 100$$

$$= \frac{716.75}{28,670} \times 100 = 2.5\%$$

Question 2: C – £1,500

Step 1: Calculate the total James will have to pay = deposit + monthly payments.

$$= (23,600 / 4) + (24 * 800) = 5,900 + 19,200 = 25,100$$

Step 2: Subtract the price from the paid price.

$$= 25,100 - 23,600 = £1,500$$

Remember the question asks about the price of the Audi A4, NOT the A5 as in the previous question.

Question 3: B – 20 miles

Step 1: Calculate the size of the petrol tank in gallons.

$$= 67.5 / 4.5 = 15$$

Step 2: Calculate how far you can drive on a third of a tank of petrol.

$$= (40 \times 15) / 3 = 600 / 3 = 200 \text{ miles}$$

Question 4: C – £35.00

Step 1: Calculate the total commute:

The total commute is the distance per day (25 miles × 2) multiplied by the number of days per week driven (5 as it states clearly in the opening section of the question) = 250 miles.

Step 2: Calculate the number of litres of petrol required.

$$= 250 / 10 = 25$$

Step 3: Calculate the total cost of petrol.

$$= 25 \times 1.40 = £35.00$$

Scenario 3

Question 1: C – 2.1 milligrams

The amount of Noradrenaline received per minute is 0.5 × 70 = 35 micrograms. Multiply this by 60 to get the amount per hour = 2,100 micrograms.

This is not an available answer. Remember your units!

1 milligrams = 1,000 micrograms, therefore 2,100 micrograms = 2.1 milligrams. Equally, looking at the answers you could quickly eliminate A and B as they are the wrong order of magnitude, as is E.

Question 2: D – 9

This is a two-step calculation. First you need to calculate how much Noradrenaline he requires per 24 hours (step 1) then work out how many syringes of DOUBLE strength Noradrenaline this is.

Step 1: 24 × 3 milligrams = 72 milligrams

Step 2: 72/8 = 9 (remember there are 8 milligrams per syringe of double strength Noradrenaline).

Question 3: E – £47.27

This is a straightforward question provided you use the right numbers. To make the solution, you will require 16 milligrams of Noradrenaline (4 vials at £11.55 each), 50 millilitres of saline (5 × 10 millilitres saline containers at £0.10 each), a syringe (£0.45) and a needle (£0.12).

The total price = (11.55 × 4) + (0.1 × 5) + 0.45 + 0.12 = £47.27.

Question 4: B – £3,285,000

Step 1: Calculate the number of 'bed nights per year'.

$= 75\%$ of $(365 \times 8) = (2,920 / 100) \times 75 = 2,190$ nights

Step 2: Calculate the total cost.

$= 2,190 \times 1,500 = £3,285,000$

Scenario 4

Question 1: D – 38.8

Reading off the chart gives us values of 40 + 36 + 60 + 32 + 26 = 194.
So the average is 194/5 = 38.8.

Question 2: C – 12.5%

Reading from the graph, we see that at Point B, in winter, flow-rate was 45 m³/s. Therefore, compared to last year it has increased by 5 m³/s.
This represents a 5/40 × 100 = 12.5% increase.

Question 3: A – 594,000

First, work out the number of seconds in two and three-quarter hours:

$2.75 \times 60 \times 60 = 9900$ seconds

Then, work out the number of metres³ that flow past in that time, using the graph information = 60 × 9,900 = 594,000 metres³. Since 1 metre³ weighs 1 tonne, this is our answer.

Question 4: D – 37.5 m³/s

At each point, flow rate increases by a factor of 1.25 between summer and winter.

For example, Point A: winter flow rate = 50 m³/s, summer flow rate = 40 m³/s. 50/40 = 1.25.

Point B: winter flow rate = 45 m³/s, summer flow rate = 36 m³/s. 45/36 = 1.25.

Therefore, from the trends on the graph, we can estimate that the flow rate at Point F will be 30 × 1.25 = 37.5 m³/s.

Scenario 5

Question 1: C – 1/5

Step 1: Work out how many blood cells make up the remaining cells other than neutrophils and leucocytes:

Total – (neutrophils + leucocytes) = 22.5 – (15.3 + 2.7) = 4.5

Step 2: Calculate the ratio: 22.5: 4.5 = 5: 1.

Question 2: B – 264

All you need to do is calculate 80% of the original platelet count of patient 3: 330/100 × 80 = 264.

Alternatively, you can quickly calculate that 10% is 33, therefore 20% is 66. 330 – 66 = 264.

Question 3: A – 624 grams

Step 1: The table tells you that the value of haemoglobin is in grams per decilitre. Remember there are 10 decilitres in 1 litre, therefore there are 60 decilitres in 6 litres (the blood volume of patient 1).

Step 2: Calculate the weight of haemoglobin: 60 × 10.4 = 624 grams.

Question 4: B – £7.00

Step 1: Calculate the cost of a 7-day course of Meropenem: (£20/2) × 3 × 7 = £210.

Step 2: Calculate the total cost of a 5-day course of Erythromycin: 210/6 = £35.

Step 3: Calculate the cost per day of Erythromycin: 35/5 = £7.

Scenario 6

Question 1: B – 73 metres^2

The total surface area is: (6 × 3) + (4 × 7) + (4 × 5) + (28/4) = 73 metres^2.

Question 2: C – 5 metres

The current kitchen is 20 metres^2, so the area of the conservatory is 10 metres^2.

The area of a semi-circle is: $(\pi r^2)/2$.

Therefore $(\pi r^2)/2 = 10$.

This gives $\pi r^2 = 20$.

$r^2 = 20/\pi = 6.37$.

Therefore $r = \sqrt{6.37} = 2.5$ metres.

Remember the diameter is twice the radius, therefore the diameter is 5 metres.

Question 3: C – £238,500

This is a simple calculation: (225,000/100) × 106 = £238,500.

Question 4: A – £46,000

There are several calculations to perform quickly.

Step 1: Calculate the deposit contributed by Archie = [(60,000/100) × 15] × 5 = £45,000.

Step 2: Calculate the total deposit placed = 340,000/5 = £68,000.

Step 3: Calculate Abbey's share = 68,000 – 45,000 = £23,000.

Step 4: Abbey's salary = 23,000/2 = £11,500 per year of contributions which is 25% of her salary. Therefore her salary = £11,500 × 4 = £46,000 per year.

Scenario 7

Question 1: A – 12,500,000

A single pellet has a volume of 3 × (3/3) × (2 × 3/3) = 6 centimetres^3.

150 metres^3 is the same as 150,000,000 centimetres^3 (1 metre = 100 centimetres, so 1 ×1 ×1 = 1 metre^3 = 100 × 100 × 100 = 1,000,000 centimetres^3).

So, 150,000,000/6 = 25,000,000 pellets are needed to fill the vat.

So, 25,000,000/2 = 12,500,000 pellets would fill half a vat.

Question 2: D – 4.8 kilograms

The volume of a single chair leg is equal to the area of the cross-sectional triangle multiplied by its length. As the area of the cross-section is given by: (*base*/2) × *height* = 5/2 × 6 = 15 centimetres^2.

So the volume of a single chair leg is given by 15 × 40 = 600 centimetres^3.

As the density of plastic is 2 g/cm^3, the mass of a single chair leg will be 2 × 600 = 1,200 grams.

As there are four chair legs, the total mass of plastic needed will be 1,200 × 4 = 4,800 grams, or 4.8 kilograms.

Question 3: D – £15,000

The cross sectional area of the triangle is (5/2) × 6 = 15 centimetres^2. The length of the prism in centimetres is given by 50 × 100 × 1,000 = 5,000,000 centimetres. That means the total volume of plastic used by the factory to make chair legs is 15 × 5,000,000 = 75,000,000 centimetres^3.

Therefore, the total mass of plastic processed is 75,000,000 × 2 = 150,000,000 grams.

As there are 1,000 kilograms in a metric tonne, that means that 150,000,000 grams = 150,000 kilograms = 150 tonnes.

So the total cost of all the plastic used will be 150 × 100 = £15,000.

Question 4: C – 1,000

We want to end up with a cabinet that weighs 10.5 kilograms (10,500 grams). We know that this final mass will be after a loss of 12.5%, so 10.5 kilograms has to equal 87.5% of the original mass of plastic put in. Therefore, the original mass will be 10.5/0.875 = 12 kilograms.

We know that a single pellet has a volume of $3 \times 1 \times 2 = 6$ centimetres^3. If the density of the plastic is 2 g/cm^3 then the mass of a single pellet is 12 grams.

Therefore we need 12,000/12 = 1,000 pellets to ensure a single cabinet can be correctly made.

Scenario 8

Question 1: C – FR$ 1319.50

If gross income in 2016 was FR$ 1,300, that means in 2017 it was $1,300 \times 1.015 = $ FR$ 1319.50, if income rose in line with inflation. Note that this figure is not over the maximum tax-free allowance threshold, so if they are only paying income tax then their gross income is the same as their income after tax deductions (because no tax is being deducted). Hence the answer is FR$ 1319.50.

Question 2: B – FR$ 9,010

The worker receives FR$ 1,300 tax-free. They are then taxed at a rate of 20% on all income up to FR$ 4,000, so they take home $0.8 \times 2,700 = $ FR$ 2,160. They are then taxed at a rate of 30% up to FR$ 10,000, so they take home $0.7 \times 6,000 = $ FR$ 4,200. They are then taxed at a rate of 40% on all income over FR$ 10,000, so they take home $0.6 \times 2,250 = $ FR$ 1,350.

Overall, $2,160 + 4,200 + 4,200 + 1,350 = $ FR$ 9,010.

Question 3: A – FR$ 6,746

A nurse gets a FR$ 1,600 allowance before paying income tax (read introduction). After that, they pay 15% on earnings up to 3,800 and take home $2,200 \times 0.85 = $ FR$ 1,870. Then they pay 22% on earnings up to FR$ 10,000 and take home $4,200 \times 0.78 = $ FR$ 3,276.

Overall, $1,600 + 1,870 + 3,276 = $ FR$ 6,746.

Question 4: D – 25.71

In 2016, a worker would have had an allowance of FR$ 1,300, would have paid 20% tax on earnings up to FR$ 4,000 ($0.2 \times 2,700 = 540$) and 30% on earnings over FR$ 4,000 but under FR$ 10,000 ($0.3 \times 1,000 = 300$). So overall tax paid was FR$ 840.

The same worker in 2017 would have had an allowance of FR$ 1,400, would have paid 15% on earnings over that up to FR$ 3,800 ($0.15 \times 2,400 = 360$) and would have paid 22% on earnings over FR$ 3,800 up to FR$ 10,000 ($0.22 \times 1,200 = 264$). So overall tax paid was FR$ 624.

Therefore, that gives a reduction of $840 - 624 = $ FR$ 216. As a percentage reduction this is $216/840 \times 100\% = 25.71\%$.

Scenario 9

Question 1: C – 0.0085 grams

Overall, we have one bull weighing 3 tonnes (3,000 kilograms), two females weighing two-thirds this (i.e. 2 × (2/3) × 3,000 = 4,000 kilograms), and three calves weighing a quarter of the weight of one female (i.e. 3 × (1/4) × 2,000 = 1,500 kilograms).

So the total elephant weight is 3,000 + 4,000 + 1,500 = 8,500 kilograms.

So we need 8,500 micrograms of *jumbodiazepane*. This is the same as 8.5 milligrams, or 0.0085 grams.

Question 2: E – 0.15 grams

An elephant weighing one and a half tonnes (1,500 kilograms) needs 1,500 micrograms of *jumbodiazepane*. Therefore, in a 10ml injection, there needs to be 1,500 micrograms of *jumbodiazepane*.

Therefore, in 1 millilitre there needs to be 150 micrograms of *jumbodiazepane*.

Therefore, in a litre batch, there needs to be 150,000 micrograms of *jumbodiazepane*, or 0.15 grams.

Question 3: B – 250

A female elephant weighs 2 tonnes (2,000 kilograms), so she needs 2,000 micrograms to send her to sleep.

If the lethal dose for a human is a tenth of a microgram per kilogram of body weight, and an average zoo vet weighs 80 kilograms, one zoo vet could be killed by 80/10 = 8 micrograms of *jumbodiazepane*.

Therefore, 2,000/8 = 250 zoo vets could be killed by the dose needed to send one female elephant to sleep.

Question 4: B – 2,500

If the lethal threshold has been lowered by a third by eating peanuts, it is now equal to 1.5 × 0.6666... = 1 microgram per kilogram of body weight.

Therefore 2.5 milligrams, or 2,500 micrograms, could kill an elephant weighing a maximum of 2,500 kilograms.

CHAPTER 4

Abstract Reasoning

Overview

Abstract Reasoning (AR) tests your ability to recognise patterns among distracting material. It does this by asking you to say whether 'test shapes' fit into certain patterns or not. The UKCAT has both static and dynamic patterns – requiring you to identify sequences and changes in patterns, before choosing which shape should come next.

Format of the Section

You will be presented with 55 questions. These need to be answered in just 14 minutes (of which 1 minute is reading time). Although this works out as just over 14 seconds per questions, many questions will be presented in sets of five. In this case, it's best to think of it as 70 seconds per question set.

There are four question types in AR:

- *Type 1*: You are presented with two 'sets' of shapes (Set A and Set B) followed by five 'test shapes'. You need to decide if the test shape fits into Set A, Set B or neither set.

- *Type 2*: This is a logical test where you are presented with a series of shapes, alternating from one box to the next. You need to say which of four shapes would come next.

- *Type 3*: This is similar to Type 2 but instead of a series you are presented with a 'statement' where changes have been applied to one shape to create a new one. You must then apply the same changes to your test shape and choose which of four options comes next.

- *Type 4*: A variation on Type 1 questions but instead of five sequential 'tests shapes' you are presented with four 'test shapes' simultaneously and have to decide which one of the four belongs to either Set A or B.

Students often find Type 2 and Type 3 questions easier than Type 1 or Type 4. This is mainly because these question types require *logical* thinking rather than pure *spatial* reasoning – a skill that scientifically and mathematically minded students prefer. The downside is that these questions tend to be far more time pressured!

Type 1 Questions

In Type 1 questions you will be presented with two sets of shapes: Set A and Set B. Each set is made up of six square boxes and each of these boxes contains a pattern. The pattern will be consistent throughout the 6 boxes in the same Set, but will be different in Set A and Set B. You will then be presented with five test shapes, one after the other, and asked if the test shape fits into Set A, Set B or neither set.

Demonstration Set

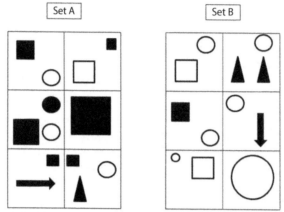

To which of the following sets do the test shapes below belong?
Test shapes:

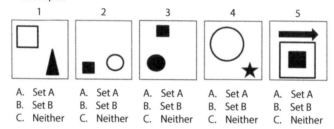

A. Set A	A. Set A	A. Set A	A. Set A	A. Set A
B. Set B	B. Set B	B. Set B	B. Set B	B. Set B
C. Neither	C. Neither	C. Neither	C. Neither	C. Neither

Answer Definitions

Set A

The test shape must match the pattern in all the boxes in Set A.

Set B

The test shape must match the pattern in all the boxes in Set B.

Neither

The test shape does *not* completely fit into either Set A or B.

OR

The test shape fits into *both* Set A and Set B (so there is no way to discriminate between the two answers).

Strategy

In order to identify the pattern and successfully answer the questions in the tight time constraint, it is essential that you stick to a strategy, adopting an efficient technique to identify the patterns.

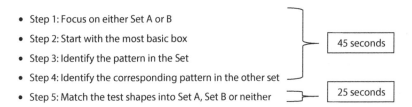

- Step 1: Focus on either Set A or B
- Step 2: Start with the most basic box
- Step 3: Identify the pattern in the Set
- Step 4: Identify the corresponding pattern in the other set

45 seconds

- Step 5: Match the test shapes into Set A, Set B or neither

25 seconds

Step 1

It doesn't matter which set you start with. Ultimately, you will need to identify the patterns in both Set A and Set B in order to match your test shapes. If you are struggling to identify the pattern in Set A, then focus on Set B. The patterns will be linked. Once you know what you're looking for (having identified the pattern in either Set A or B), you can apply those same rules to the opposite set. Hopefully, it should be easy to identify the second pattern.

Step 2

Identifying the pattern can be challenging. So here's a basic first trick to help you along. When assessing either Set A or B, look for the box containing the least number of items, in other words, the most basic box. Remember, the pattern has to be present in all six boxes of a set. It is easier to identify the pattern if there are fewer items to process.

Start by finding the most basic box in each set:

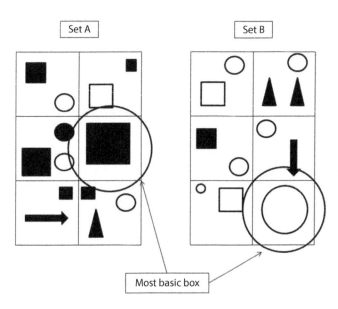

Most basic box

The earlier is a simplified example. It demonstrates that finding the pattern is much easier when there are fewer items to assess. However, this technique has two limiting factors:

1. What if there is no 'most basic' box?

2. You might still not be able to identify the pattern.

Steps 3 and 4

Identifying the pattern(s) is the most challenging part of the question. There seems to be infinite possible combinations. However, certain themes are more common than others. Patterns can be categorised in two ways:

- Non-conditional
- Conditional

Non-conditional patterns occur when the themes are independent and do not depend on each other. Common examples include number of items, sides, angles, intersections, etc. There may be several non-conditional patterns present in each set, but they are intrinsically linked between Set A and Set B (otherwise, it would be impossible to identify all patterns in just 45 seconds).

Conditional patterns occur when one of the themes is dependent on another. Students often find these tricky. For instance, the pattern might be: if the triangle points up in Set A, then there will be an odd number of small squares in the box; if it points down, then the number of small squares is even.

In Type 1 questions, you have just over 70 seconds per question set. You should therefore allow yourself up to 45 seconds to identify the patterns in Set A and B. This leaves you with 25 seconds to match your test shapes to the correct set.

It is imperative that you keep an eye on the timer! If you have not found the pattern within 45 seconds, you must select answers according to your gut instinct, 'flag' the question, and move on. Otherwise, you risk running out of time to complete the AR section. If you have time to spare after completing the section, you can then attempt flagged questions again.

Step 5

Once you have identified the patterns in Set A and Set B, it is relatively quick to match your test shapes with the correct set. The process of assessing the test shape, matching it to the correct set and moving to the next question should take around 5 seconds.

> **Top Tip:** Keep a close eye on the clock. It's easy to get bogged down looking for a pattern and losing valuable time.

Distractors

Abstract reasoning involves identifying patterns which are disguised among superfluous material. Within the boxes, there are often numerous items which do not contribute to the overall pattern. Rather, they *mask* the pattern by 'distracting' you. These are the so-called 'distractors'. Until you know what the pattern is, you will not be able to identify which items are distractors and which contribute to the actual pattern. Distractors can therefore make it significantly harder to identify the underlying pattern.

Once you know what the pattern is, you can identify which items are distractors. In the following example, the simple pattern is a shaded square in every box of Set A. With this in mind, you can appreciate the distractors at work.

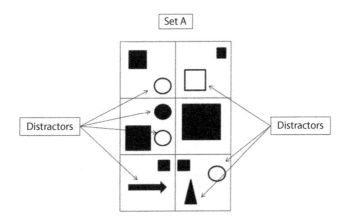

Troubleshooting

You might have trouble finding the pattern. In which case, try the following:

1. Move around! Some patterns are easier to see close up. Others are more obvious the further away you are. 'Big picture' patterns, such as position and colour distribution, are easy to overlook when sitting close to the screen. So, if you're struggling, it is a good idea to move around and change your perspective.

2. Focus on both sets. The patterns between Set A and Set B are linked. Therefore, if you can't find the pattern in Set A, focus on Set B. Once you have identified a pattern in one set, you can apply the theme to the other. Hopefully, you will then find the pattern easily.

3. If you still can't find the pattern and you have used your 45 seconds then you must *move on*. It is easy to become engrossed in finding patterns. Before you know it several minutes can pass. This makes it impossible to finish the rest of the section in time.

Patterns

There are a wide range of potential patterns. But there are a few common patterns that crop up regularly. Although it seems tough, students often report that Abstract Reasoning was the only section of the exam that was easier than expected!

Examples of common patterns include:

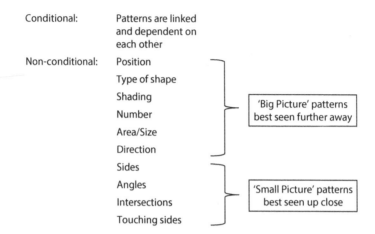

Conditional: Patterns are linked and dependent on each other

Non-conditional: Position
Type of shape
Shading
Number
Area/Size
Direction

'Big Picture' patterns best seen further away

Sides
Angles
Intersections
Touching sides

'Small Picture' patterns best seen up close

Top Tip: An anagram to help you look for common patterns is TITANS PADS:

- **T**ype of shape
- **I**ntersections
- **T**ouching sides
- **A**rea and size
- **N**umber
- **S**hading
- **P**osition
- **A**ngles
- **D**irection
- **S**ides

It is advisable to look for at least two patterns per set. Although there will be some difficult questions, which may feature more patterns, finding at least two patterns will allow you to get the correct answer in the majority of questions. After you have identified what the pattern relates to – e.g. right angles – you need to figure out how exactly it works. Considering the following three possibilities will help with this process:

- Absolutes numbers: What is the absolute number of a particular item/theme in each set?
- Odd/Even: Is there an odd number of a particular theme in one set, and an even number in the other?
- Greater or Lesser than: Is the pattern simply that there are more than or less than a specific number of a particular item/theme in each set?

> **Top Tip:** If you spot a pattern falling into the odd/even category, always consider the possibility of a second pattern being present. Otherwise, the pattern would be too simple and 'neither' may never be a viable answer option depending on the pattern.

The Impression Technique

When you first look at a question, there are a number of different 'impressions' you might get. Broadly speaking, these fall into seven categories. For each impression there are a number of commonly occurring patterns to look for. Although there are exceptions, the majority of the time if you know what you're looking for, suddenly the 'hunt' becomes much easier. Memorising what to look for in each impression will help you perform a structured search of the most commonly occurring patterns.

We have divided the impressions into seven categories:

- 'Everything looks the same'
- 'Different shapes'
- 'Arrows by themselves'
- 'Letters and Words'
- 'Familiar objects'
- 'Abstract patterns'
- 'Something's changing'

In addition to the earlier, there are also three *Special Circumstances* where rarely occurring events will offer clues to the correct pattern:

- Items touching the side
- Items overlapping
- Arrows pointing to/from items

We will now work our way through numerous examples, looking at the different impressions and the potential patterns with which they associate. Refer to the following *Example Set 1*. Set a timer for 70 seconds and make a note of your answers before moving on to the explanations.

Example Set 1

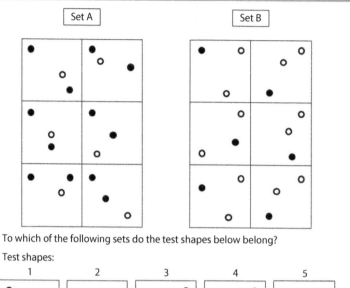

To which of the following sets do the test shapes below belong?

Test shapes:

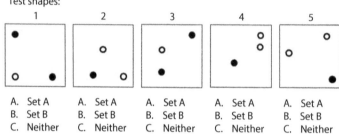

1	2	3	4	5
A. Set A	A. Set A	A. Set A	A. Set A	A. Set A
B. Set B	B. Set B	B. Set B	B. Set B	B. Set B
C. Neither	C. Neither	C. Neither	C. Neither	C. Neither

Example Set 1: Answers and Explanations

In this set there are two patterns: position and shading. Both are 'big picture' patterns and easier to see the farther away from the sets you are. In Set A, there are 2 shaded circles and one unshaded circle in every box, with one shaded circle in the top-left-hand corner. In Set B, there are two unshaded circles and one shaded circle in each box, with one unshaded circle in the top-right-hand corner.

Test Shape 1: Set A – There are two shaded circles and one unshaded circle, with one shaded circle in the top-left-hand corner.

Test Shape 2: Neither – Although it has two unshaded circles and one shaded circle, there is no unshaded circle in the top-right-hand corner.

Test Shape 3: Neither – It has the colour distribution for Set A but the position (albeit the wrong shading) for Set B.

Test Shape 4: Set B – There are two unshaded circles, one of which is in the top-right-hand corner and one shaded circle.

Test Shape 5: Set B – Same as earlier.

Top Tip: If there is more than one pattern present, the question will usually be designed in such a way that spotting one pattern will still score you some points.

Impression 1 – Everything Looks the Same

Sometimes you are faced with two sets that look almost identical. There are relatively few patterns that commonly fit this scenario. This is due to the fact that many patterns will cancel themselves out when the two sets use the same item number and type in each box. The main patterns to look for when everything looks the same are:

- Position
- Shading
- Conditional

If you failed to spot both patterns in this example, then look back now. Hopefully you will find it much easier now that you know what to look for. Try to apply this in the future when faced with near identical looking sets.

Refer to the following *Example Set 2*. Set a timer for 70 seconds and make a note of your answers before moving on to the explanations.

Example Set 2

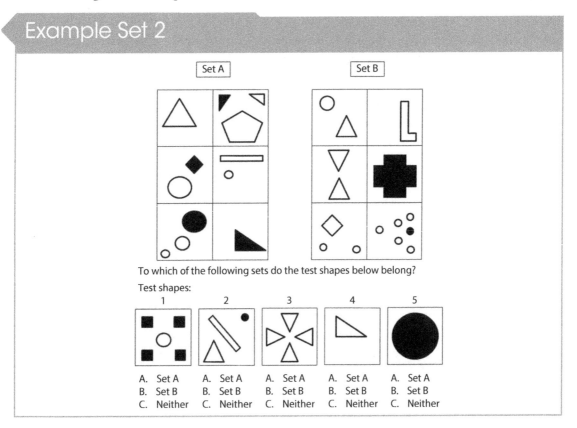

To which of the following sets do the test shapes below belong?

Test shapes:

1	2	3	4	5
A. Set A	A. Set A	A. Set A	A. Set A	A. Set A
B. Set B	B. Set B	B. Set B	B. Set B	B. Set B
C. Neither	C. Neither	C. Neither	C. Neither	C. Neither

Example Set 2: Answers and Explanations

There is only one pattern in this set: the total number of sides in every box. In Set A, the total number of sides is an odd number. In Set B, it is an even number. Remember that a circle has 1 side (not an infinite number of sides, as so many students mistakenly assume). In this case, there is no pattern in terms of shading. The shading merely acts as a distractor.

> **Top Tip:** If you only identify an odd/even pattern then it's important that you look for a second pattern. Otherwise 'neither' may not be a viable answer option.

Test Shape 1: Set A – 17 sides in total

Test Shape 2: Set B – 8 sides in total

Test Shape 3: Set B – 12 sides in total

Test Shape 4: Set A – 3 sides in total

Test Shape 5: Set A – 1 side in total

Impression 2 – Different Shapes

Seeing boxes comprising seemingly random shapes can be daunting. It's difficult to know where to begin. Unfortunately, sets consisting of different shapes do lend themselves to numerous potential patterns. There are seven patterns to look for in this situation. Six are common and one is a rare pattern:

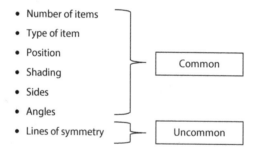

- Number of items
- Type of item
- Position
- Shading
- Sides
- Angles

Common

- Lines of symmetry

Uncommon

The most common angles-based patterns use right angles. If you see right-angled shapes in every box then it is worth counting the number looking for an absolute, or an odd/even pattern.

> **Top Tip:** When faced with random shapes there are a lot of potential patterns to look for. If you see only circles, then you can eliminate 'angles' and 'lines of symmetry'.

Refer to the following *Example Set 3*. Set a timer for 70 seconds and make a note of your answers before moving on to the explanations.

Example Set 3

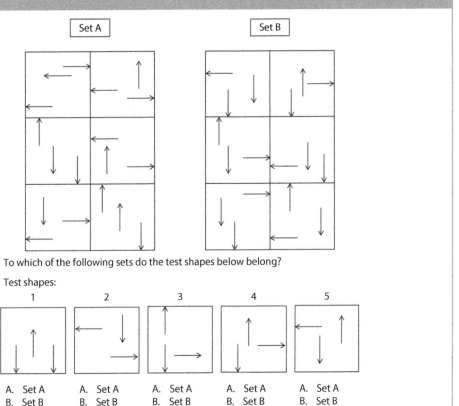

Set A   Set B

To which of the following sets do the test shapes below belong?

Test shapes:

1	2	3	4	5

A. Set A   A. Set A   A. Set A   A. Set A   A. Set A
B. Set B   B. Set B   B. Set B   B. Set B   B. Set B
C. Neither   C. Neither   C. Neither   C. Neither   C. Neither

Example Set 3: Answers and Explanations

In of these sets, all you have is arrows! Each box – in both Set A and Set B – contains three arrows in total, two of which touch the sides. In Set A, the arrows always touch opposite sides. In Set B, however, they touch adjacent sides. There is no other pattern present.

Test Shape 1: Neither – There are two arrows touching sides but they both touch the same side.

Test Shape 2: Set A – There are two arrows touching opposite sides.

Test Shape 3: Set A – There are two arrows touching opposite sides.

Test Shape 4: Set B – There are two arrows touching adjacent sides.

Test Shape 5: Neither – There is only one arrow touching a side.

Impression 3 – Arrows by Themselves

Doing an Abstract Reasoning question based entirely on arrows can be overwhelming. The reality is that there are actually quite a limited number of potential patterns that could be present. If all you see are arrows, then the four main patterns to look out for are:

- Number
- Direction
- Position
- Touching Sides

Special Circumstances – Touching Sides

It is unusual for shapes to touch the sides of the boxes in abstract reasoning. If you see shapes consistently touching sides then always assess this before looking for other patterns. When items touch sides, there are several possible patterns, depending on:

- Which side(s) is being touched
- The number of sides being touched

Refer to the following *Example Set 4*. Set a timer for 70 seconds and make a note of your answers before moving on to the explanations.

Example Set 4

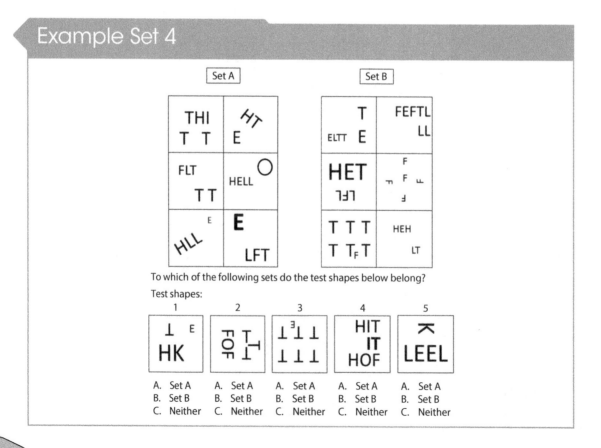

Example Set 4: Answers and Explanations

When seeing a set of questions consisting of words and letters, it is important to remember that these are, in fact, not words and letters per se. Instead, you should view them simply as abstract shapes (that just happen to resemble words and letters). Abstract reasoning is assessing your ability to identify physical patterns. So, any meaning attributed to the shapes does not contribute towards the pattern. In the aforementioned example, there is only one pattern present: There are 10 right angles per box in Set A, and 15 right angles per box in set B. The capital letters E, F, H, L and T are all made up of right angles (E = 4, F = 3, H = 4, L = 1 and T = 2).

> Test Shape 1: Set A – 10 right angles
>
> Test Shape 2: Neither – 12 right angles
>
> Test Shape 3: Neither – 16 right angles
>
> Test Shape 4: Set B – 15 right angles
>
> Test Shape 5: Set A – 10 right angles

Impression 4 – Letters and Words

Although they look complex, questions involving letters or words are still only assessing the *physical properties* of the 'shapes'. The patterns never relate to meaning. Certain letters (E, F, H, L and T) lend themselves to right angles. So when these letters are present, you must always consider this pattern first. The patterns you should look for when presented with letters and words are:

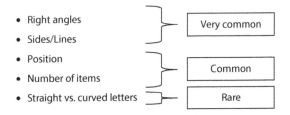

As you are only assessing the physical properties of the shapes – and not the meaning – you should not routinely consider the following as part of a pattern:

- Upper versus Lower Case
- Vowel versus Consonant
- Meaning of the words

Refer to the following *Example Set 5*. Set a timer for 70 seconds and make a note of your answers before moving on to the explanations.

Example Set 5

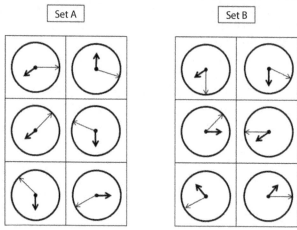

Set A   Set B

To which of the following sets do the test shapes below belong?

Test shapes:

1   2   3   4   5

A. Set A	A. Set A	A. Set A	A. Set A	A. Set A
B. Set B	B. Set B	B. Set B	B. Set B	B. Set B
C. Neither	C. Neither	C. Neither	C. Neither	C. Neither

Example Set 5: Answers and Explanations

The previous picture set presents you with a series of 'clocks'. Although, as with all abstract reasoning, they are not truly clocks. Rather, they are combinations of shapes that resemble clocks! The most striking feature you will notice when faced with clock faces are the angles. Although angles are likely to play a part, don't forget to assess the shapes for other physical properties. In this case, both sets contain a large circle, within which there is a long thin arrow which connects with the circle, and a short fat arrow – which does not. In Set A, the angle between the two arrows is obtuse (>90°). In Set B, the angle between the two arrows is acute (<90°).

    Test Shape 1: Set B – There is an acute angle between the arrows.

    Test Shape 2: Neither – There is a right angle between the arrows, so as a result the angle is neither acute nor obtuse between the arrows.

Abstract Reasoning

Test Shape 3: Set A – There is an obtuse angle between the arrows.

Test Shape 4: Neither – There is an obtuse angle between the arrows, so the test shape initially appears to belong to Set A. However, the long thin arrow does not connect with the circle, and therefore the physical properties are different.

Test Shape 5: Set A – There is an obtuse angle between the arrows.

Impression 5 – Familiar Objects

The objects in Set A and Set B may mimic 'familiar' objects, such as clocks, dominoes, or even faces. But they must nevertheless be assessed on the basis of their *physical properties*. The more familiar the object, the easier it is to overlook this crucial point. In the previous example, it is easy to make a mistake on test shape 4, where the angle fits with Set A but physical properties differ.

'Clocks' can be presented both as analogue and digital displays. It is crucial to remember that 'time' itself cannot be a pattern. So, having morning vs. evening, for instance, wouldn't work.

Example of a digital clock display:

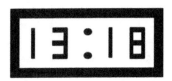

Although the time itself cannot be a pattern, different times will generate different potential patterns. This might include the number of lines or, in the previous image, the number of right angles.

Refer to the following *Example Set 6*. Set a timer for 70 seconds and make a note of your answers before moving on to the explanations.

Example Set 6

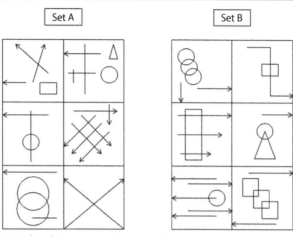

To which of the following sets do the test shapes below belong?

Test shapes:

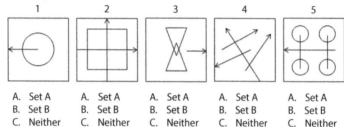

1	2	3	4	5
A. Set A	A. Set A	A. Set A	A. Set A	A. Set A
B. Set B	B. Set B	B. Set B	B. Set B	B. Set B
C. Neither	C. Neither	C. Neither	C. Neither	C. Neither

Example Set 6: Answers and Explanations

In this question set there are two patterns: intersections and touching sides. In Set A, there are an odd number of intersections. But remember: whenever faced with an odd/even pattern you must always look for a second pattern. In this case, there is also an arrow touching the left side of every box. In Set B, there are an even number of intersections – and an arrow touching the right side of every box. Touching sides is an unusual pattern so whenever you see shapes or objects touching the side of the box, always explore this for a pattern (even if other patterns appear obvious).

Test Shape 1: Set A – There is an odd number of intersections and an arrow touching the left.

Test Shape 2: Neither – There is an odd number of intersections but no arrow touching the left.

Test Shape 3: Set B – There is an even number of intersections and an arrow touching the right.

Test Shape 4: Set A – There is an odd number of intersections and an arrow touching the left.

Test Shape 5: Neither – There is an even number of intersections but no arrow touching the right.

Impression 6 – Abstract Patterns

When faced with the apparent randomness of anything from shapes, lines and arrows through to 'squiggly lines', then you must always consider:

- Number of items
- Intersections
- Touching sides
- Angles
- Areas

Special Circumstances – Items Overlapping

It is unusual for items to be placed on top of each other. If they are, this creates crossing points known as intersections. Whenever you see this occurring, consider whether this is your underlying pattern.

Top Tip: The point at which a shape touches the side of a box is not an intersection, as technically it does not cross over. So, do not count 'touching sides' as intersections.

Refer to the following *Example Set 7*. Set a timer for 70 seconds and make a note of your answers before moving on to the explanations.

Example Set 7

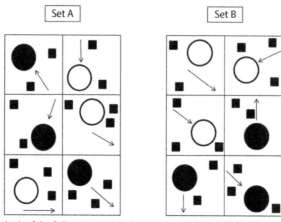

To which of the following sets do the test shapes below belong?

Test shapes:

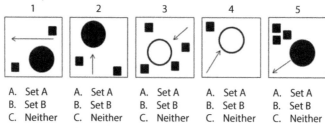

1	2	3	4	5
A. Set A	A. Set A	A. Set A	A. Set A	A. Set A
B. Set B	B. Set B	B. Set B	B. Set B	B. Set B
C. Neither	C. Neither	C. Neither	C. Neither	C. Neither

Example Set 7: Answers and Explanations

This is our first example of a conditional pattern. These occur when the patterns are linked and dependent upon each other. When dealing with conditional patterns, ask yourself: 'If X happens to Y, what happens to Z?' In the earlier set, you can see that there are arrows either pointing towards the circle or away from it. So, the question is: what happens when the arrow points towards/away from the circle? In Set A, when the arrow points towards the circle there are two squares in each box; when it points away, there are three squares. In Set B, when the arrow points towards the circle there are three squares in each box; when the arrow points away, there are two squares. There is no pattern relating to the position of the squares or shading of the circle.

Test Shape 1: Set B – The arrow points away from the circle and there are two squares.

Test Shape 2: Set A – The arrow points towards the circle and there are two squares.

Test Shape 3: Neither – There are four squares in the test box, which doesn't fit with Set A or B.

Test Shape 4: Neither – There is only one square in the test box, which doesn't fit with the pattern in either Set A or B.

Test Shape 5: Set A – The arrow points away from the circle and there are three squares in the box.

Impression 7 – Something's Changing

You look at Set A and Set B. They appear to be very similar. Yet something seems to keep changing. In that case, it's almost certainly a conditional question. Conditional patterns are linked and dependent on each other. In this case, you need to look at the boxes in detail and ascertain which components are changing, and how. By doing so, you can figure out the conditional pattern. The five things that are most likely to change in conditional questions are:

- Number of items
- Position
- Shading
- Size of items
- Direction

Special Circumstances – Arrows Pointing to/from Items

If you encounter a question set containing arrows which point either to or from items then this is almost certainly a conditional question. So, your next task is to identify what other patterns arise when the direction of the arrow changes.

Refer to the following *Example Set 8*. Set a timer for 70 seconds and make a note of your answers before moving on to the explanations.

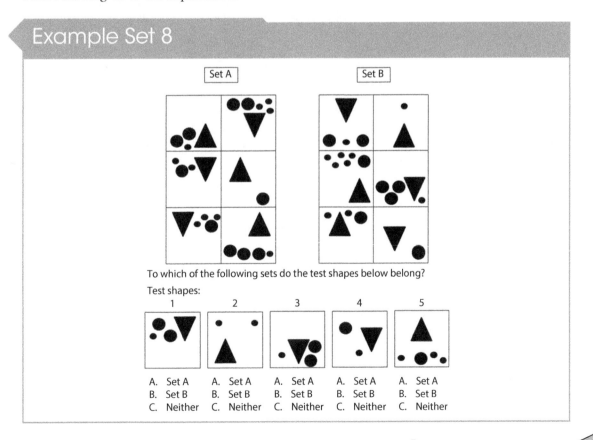

Example Set 8: Answers and Explanations

This is another example of a conditional pattern. But this time there are two conditional patterns present: size and position.

In Set A, if the triangle points up, then the circles are in the bottom half of the box and there are more large circles than small ones. If the triangle points down, then the circles are in top half of the box and there are more small circles than large ones.

The pattern in Set B is the opposite. If the triangle points up, then the circles are in the top half of the box and there are more small circles than large ones. If the triangle points down, then the circles are in the bottom half of the box and there are more large circles than small ones.

Test Shape 1: Neither – The triangle points down and the circles are in the top half. But there are more large circles than small ones. Therefore, the position of the circles is in keeping with Set A – but the size distribution is in keeping with Set B.

Test Shape 2: Set B – The triangle points up and the circles are in the top half of the box, with more small circles than large ones.

Test Shape 3: Set B – The triangle points down and the circles are in the bottom half of the box, with more large circles than small ones.

Test Shape 4: Neither – There are circles in both halves of the box which is not in keeping with either Set A or B.

Test Shape 5: Neither – The triangle points up and the circles are in the bottom half. But there are more small circles than large ones. Therefore, the position fits with Set A but the size distribution fits with Set B.

Top Tips for Type 1 Questions

1. *Change your perspective* (move closer and farther away from the computer screen) to ensure you see both small and big picture patterns.

2. If you can't identify the pattern within *45 seconds* go with your gut instinct, flag the question and *move on*.

3. Always look for *two patterns*, especially if you spot an odd/even distribution, as there is usually a second pattern also present.

4. Use the *Impression Technique* to quickly narrow down what patterns to look for and what to eliminate.

5. Remember the three *special circumstances*: touching sides, overlapping shapes and arrows pointing to/from items. These rare events often allow you to quickly identify the underlying pattern.

Additional Question Formats

In addition to type 1 questions, there are three other question styles in the Abstract Reasoning component of the UKCAT exam: Type 2, Type 3 and Type 4.

The Type 2 and 3 questions are 'dynamic' questions. Unlike Type 1 and 4 questions, where you need to identify a fixed pattern and match test shapes accordingly, Type 2 and 3 questions feature a changing pattern. Luckily, students often find it easier to identify this dynamic change, as opposed to static patterns. The main difficulty with Type 2 and 3 questions is the short time limit.

Students may have encountered similar question styles to type 2 and 3 questions in the past. They are a staple of many IQ and career aptitude tests.

Type 2 Questions

In Type 2 questions, you are presented with a series of four boxes of shapes. Changes occur from one box to the next. Your task is to identify what, exactly, is changing and to decide which of four options would come next in the sequence. The time pressure with this question type is significant. You have just under 15 seconds per question, so you must stick ruthlessly to your strategy.

Strategy for Type 2 Questions

1. Break the items in each box into individual 'components'.

2. Focus on one component at a time, looking at how it changes from one box to the next and paying close attention to:

   - Position
   - Shading
   - Direction/Rotation
   - Size

3. As you assess each component in turn, eliminate answer options which don't fit with the next anticipated change.

4. Using this technique, you will eliminate answer options one by one until only the correct answer remains.

Refer to the following *Example Sets 9 to 11*. Set a timer for *45 seconds* and make a note of your answers before moving on to the explanations.

Example Set 9

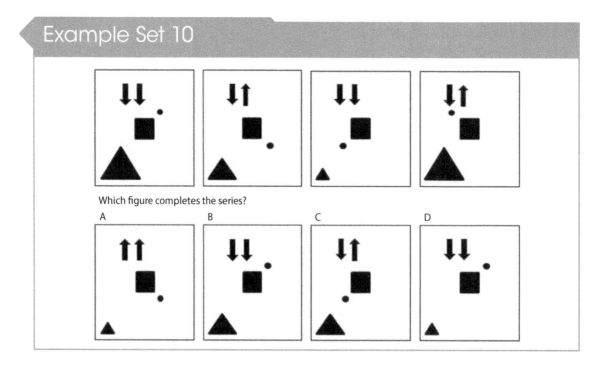

Which figure completes the series?

Example Set 10

Which figure completes the series?

Example Set 11

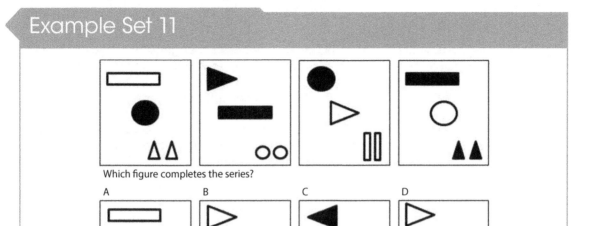

Which figure completes the series?

A   B   C   D

Example Sets 9 to 11: Answers and Explanations

Set 9 – Option C

There are four components to this shape: a central three pronged spoke, a triangle, and a black and a white square. The central spoke rotates clockwise 90° between each box. So, this allows you to eliminate option A. The triangle alternates between pointing towards the spoke and away from it. So, you can also eliminate options A and D. Both the black and white square move in the same way between the boxes: from the top, to the middle, to the bottom, then back to the top again. Looking at the white square alone allows you to eliminate option B. Looking at the black square allows you to eliminate A and D. It doesn't matter which component you begin. But you can often reach the correct answer through elimination, without having to assess every aspect.

Set 10 – Option B

There are many changing elements in this set: a central square with an associated black circle which rotates 90° each time; a triangle in the bottom-left corner which changes size from large to medium to small then back to large again; and a combination of two arrows, where the right-hand arrow alternates between pointing down and up, and the left-hand arrow is static and pointing down. Applying these rules allows us to see the only possible answer is B.

Set 11 – Option D

Again, this question features a number of patterns that keep changing. Firstly, the position of the items changes so that the item in the top-left corner moves to the middle, then the bottom-right-hand corner, before returning to the top left. Secondly, when the item reaches the bottom-right-hand corner, it divides into two identical but smaller copies, which rotate 90° clockwise. The item then returns to its original size and number when moving back into the top-left-hand corner. Finally, the shading of each item alternates between shaded and unshaded. After the process of elimination, only answer option D remains.

Type 3 Questions

Like Type 2 questions, Type 3 questions assess your ability to identify a dynamic pattern. You are given two shapes that somehow relate to each other. You will then be given a third shape, and asked which one of four options would, by the same logic, relate to that. The time pressure is once again intense, with just under 15 seconds available per question. So, strategy and stamina are essential.

Strategy for Type 3 Questions

The strategy employed for Type 3 questions is similar to that used for Type 2:

1. Focus on the individual components of the example box, one by one.

2. Identify which components have changed and which have remained static.

3. These static components must also remain static in your new test box.

4. Identify and apply the dynamic changes to your test shape, eliminating answers options that don't match until you are left with the correct answer.

Refer to the following *Example Sets 12 and 13*. Set a timer for *30 seconds* and make a note of your answers before moving on to the explanations.

Example Set 12

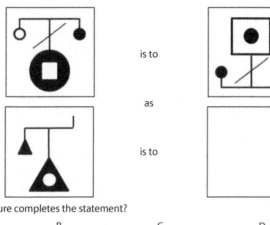

is to

as

is to

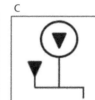

Which figure completes the statement?

A   B   C   D

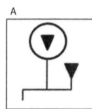 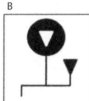 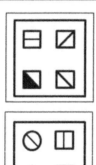

Example Set 13

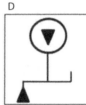

is to

as

is to

Which figure completes the statement?

A   B   C   D

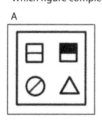 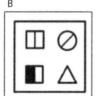 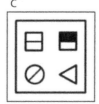 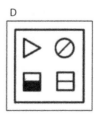

Example Sets 12 and 13: Answers and Explanations

Set 12 – Option A

Rotation and direction are particularly important in Type 3 questions. Looking at the demonstration set shows you that the entire structure rotates 180° clockwise. You can quickly deduce this, as the position of the shaded and unshaded circles swaps around while the intersecting straight line remains upward sloping. If it had inverted, then the position of the shaded and unshaded circles would have remained the same, while the angle of the intersecting straight line would have become downward sloping. The second change is that the circle and square swap size and position (but not shading).

When you apply these rules to your test shape, you will see that Option A fits the aforementioned rules. In Option B, the circle and triangle have swapped shading as well as size and position, which is incorrect. Option C would fit with inversion, not rotation. And Option D is not viable, as the triangle has moved to the outside of the structure.

Set 13 – Option C

This kind of combination of shapes can be quite confusing at first. But if you look at the structure contained within the square as a whole, you will notice that the only change is that the entire structure has rotated 90° anti-clockwise. There are no further changes taking place to any of the smaller shapes within the square.

In Option A, the problem lies with the triangle: the direction is wrong. If the triangle had rotated 90° anti-clockwise, it would point towards the circle – as in the correct answer, Option C. Option B is incorrect as it is the result of a side-to-side inversion. In Option D, the whole structure has rotated 90° clockwise – instead of anti-clockwise.

Type 4 Questions

Type 4 questions are, in essence, almost identical to Type 1. They are just more time pressured! You will be presented with two sets of shapes: Set A and Set B. This time, however, you do not get a series of test shapes you need to match to one set or another. Instead, you are presented with four test shapes simultaneously and asked one of two questions:

- Which of the following test shapes belongs in Set A?

    OR

- Which of the following test shapes belongs in Set B?

So, you need to utilise precisely the same skills employed when answering Type 1 questions, in order to identify the pattern in Sets A and Set B. This will allow you to answer either of the questions posed earlier.

Time for some practice! Try answering the following *11 Practice Sets* containing *55 questions*. There is a mixture of type 1, 2, 3 and 4 questions. You have 14 minutes to answer all questions. Detailed explanations are provided. Good luck!

Questions

Question Set 1

| Set A | Set B |

To which of the following sets do the test shapes below belong?

Test shapes:

| 1 | 2 | 3 | 4 | 5 |

1	2	3	4	5
A. Set A	A. Set A	A. Set A	A. Set A	A. Set A
B. Set B	B. Set B	B. Set B	B. Set B	B. Set B
C. Neither	C. Neither	C. Neither	C. Neither	C. Neither

Question Set 2

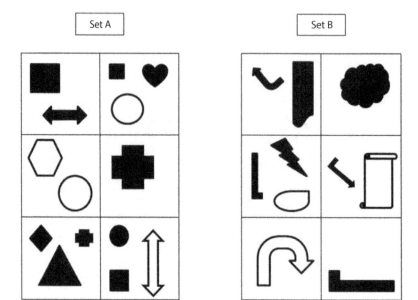

To which of the following sets do the test shapes below belong?

Test shapes:

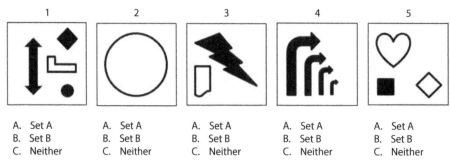

1	2	3	4	5
A. Set A	A. Set A	A. Set A	A. Set A	A. Set A
B. Set B	B. Set B	B. Set B	B. Set B	B. Set B
C. Neither	C. Neither	C. Neither	C. Neither	C. Neither

Question Set 3

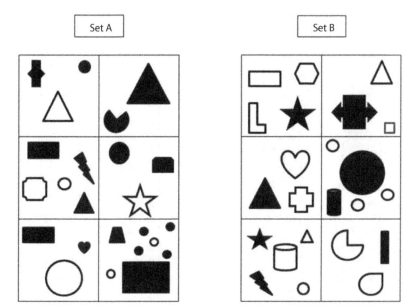

To which of the following sets do the test shapes below belong?

Test shapes:

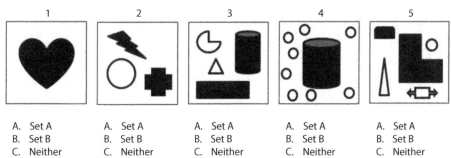

1	2	3	4	5
A. Set A	A. Set A	A. Set A	A. Set A	A. Set A
B. Set B	B. Set B	B. Set B	B. Set B	B. Set B
C. Neither	C. Neither	C. Neither	C. Neither	C. Neither

Question Set 4

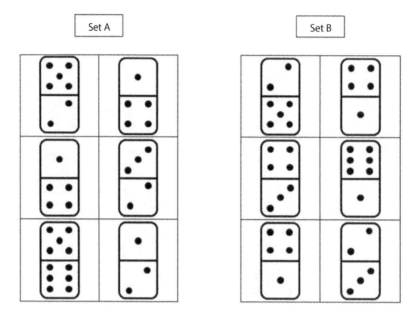

To which of the following sets do the test shapes below belong?

Test shapes:

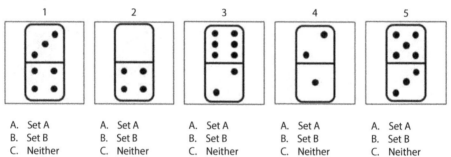

1	2	3	4	5
A. Set A	A. Set A	A. Set A	A. Set A	A. Set A
B. Set B	B. Set B	B. Set B	B. Set B	B. Set B
C. Neither	C. Neither	C. Neither	C. Neither	C. Neither

Question Set 5

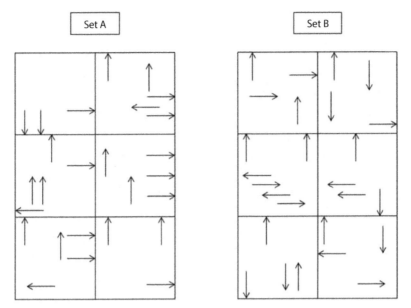

To which of the following sets do the test shapes below belong?

Test shapes:

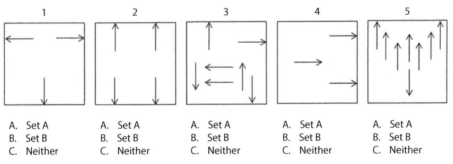

1	2	3	4	5
A. Set A	A. Set A	A. Set A	A. Set A	A. Set A
B. Set B	B. Set B	B. Set B	B. Set B	B. Set B
C. Neither	C. Neither	C. Neither	C. Neither	C. Neither

Question Set 6

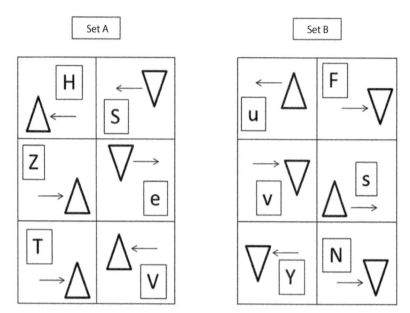

To which of the following sets do the test shapes below belong?

Test shapes:

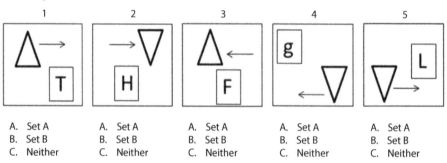

1	2	3	4	5
A. Set A	A. Set A	A. Set A	A. Set A	A. Set A
B. Set B	B. Set B	B. Set B	B. Set B	B. Set B
C. Neither	C. Neither	C. Neither	C. Neither	C. Neither

Question Set 7

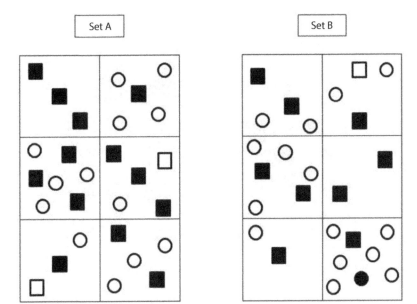

Set A   Set B

To which of the following sets do the test shapes below belong?

Test shapes:

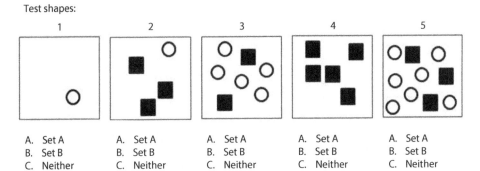

1
A. Set A
B. Set B
C. Neither

2
A. Set A
B. Set B
C. Neither

3
A. Set A
B. Set B
C. Neither

4
A. Set A
B. Set B
C. Neither

5
A. Set A
B. Set B
C. Neither

Question Set 8

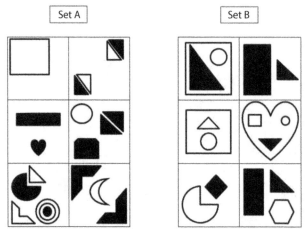

To which of the following sets do the test shapes below belong?

Test shapes:

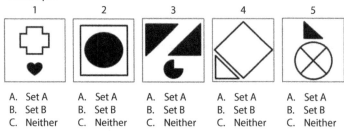

1	2	3	4	5
A. Set A	A. Set A	A. Set A	A. Set A	A. Set A
B. Set B	B. Set B	B. Set B	B. Set B	B. Set B
C. Neither	C. Neither	C. Neither	C. Neither	C. Neither

Question Set 9 – Question 1

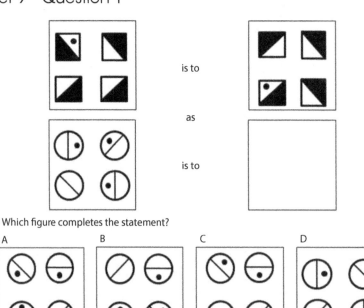

is to

as

is to

Which figure completes the statement?

A   B   C   D

Question Set 9 – Question 2

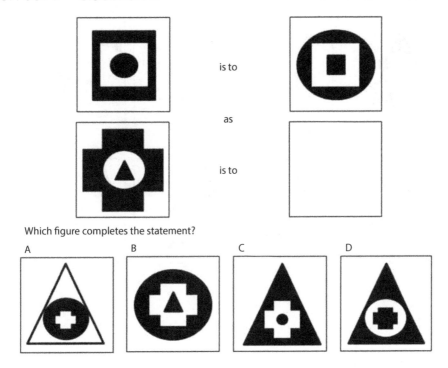

Which figure completes the statement?

Question Set 9 – Question 3

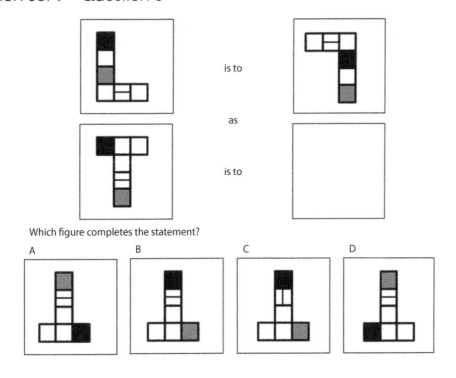

Which figure completes the statement?

Question Set 9 – Question 4

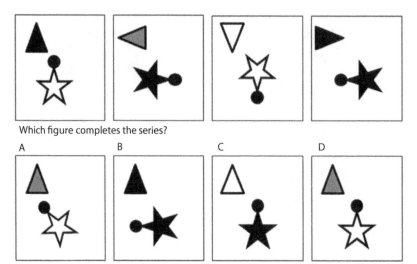

Which figure completes the series?

A   B   C   D

Question Set 9 – Question 5

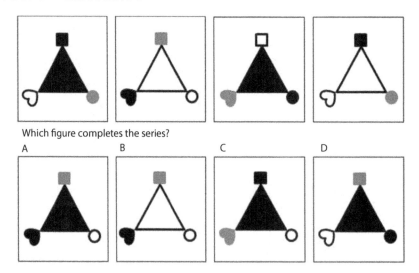

Which figure completes the series?

A   B   C   D

Question Set 10

Set A   Set B

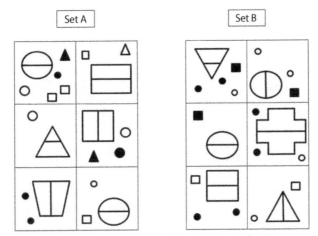

To which of the following sets do the test shapes below belong?

Test shapes:

1   2   3   4   5

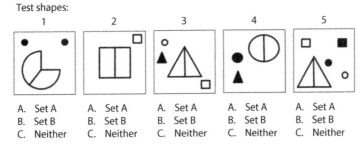

A. Set A	A. Set A	A. Set A	A. Set A	A. Set A
B. Set B	B. Set B	B. Set B	B. Set B	B. Set B
C. Neither	C. Neither	C. Neither	C. Neither	C. Neither

Question Set 11

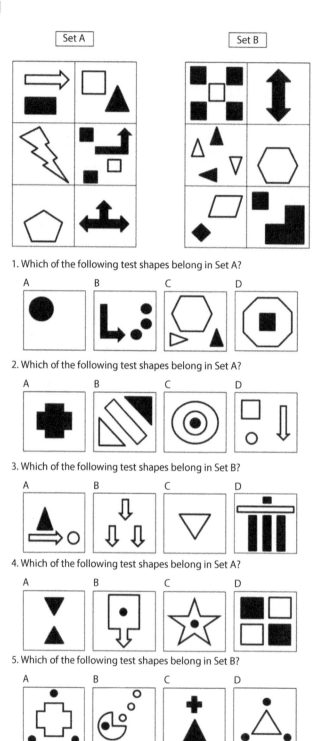

1. Which of the following test shapes belong in Set A?

A   B   C   D

2. Which of the following test shapes belong in Set A?

A   B   C   D

3. Which of the following test shapes belong in Set B?

A   B   C   D

4. Which of the following test shapes belong in Set A?

A   B   C   D

5. Which of the following test shapes belong in Set B?

A   B   C   D

Answers

Question Set 1

This question is relatively straight forward and is looking at the position of objects. In Set A there is an upward facing curved arrow in the top-left corner of each box, whilst in set B there is a downward facing curved arrow in the top-left corner of each box.

Test Shape 1: Neither

Test Shape 2: Set B

Test Shape 3: Set A

Test Shape 4: Set A

Test Shape 5: Set B

Question Set 2

This question is quite tricky, but again, is only testing one theme – symmetry. In set A, all the shapes are symmetrical whereas in set B they are not.

Test Shape 1: Neither (as it is a mix of symmetrical and non-symmetrical shapes)

Test Shape 2: Set A

Test Shape 3: Set B

Test Shape 4: Set B

Test Shape 5: Set A

Question Set 3

This question set contains boxes which contain seemingly similar shapes with no obvious pattern. The pattern present is that in Set A there are always more shaded than non-shaded shapes in each box, with the reverse true for Set B.

Test Shape 1: Set A

Test Shape 2: Set A

Test Shape 3: Neither

Test Shape 4: Set B

Test Shape 5: Set B

Question Set 4

In this question you are faced with Dominoes, but again remember to treat them as shapes and look for the same types of pattern as you would normally. In set A there is an odd number on top with an even number below, with the reverse pattern in set B.

Test Shape 1: Set A

Test Shape 2: Neither

Test Shape 3: Neither

Test Shape 4: Set B

Test Shape 5: Neither

Question Set 5

This question is hard as it is looking at various themes simultaneously. In set A, there is always an odd number of arrows in total, with 3 arrows touching sides in every box and an arrow touching the right-hand side of the box in every shape. In set B, there is an even total number of arrows, an arrow touching the top side of each box and a total of 2 arrows touching sides in each box.

Test Shape 1: Set A

Test Shape 2: Neither

Test Shape 3: Set A

Test Shape 4: Neither

Test Shape 5: Set B

Question Set 6

This question is difficult. There are several themes to spot, including a conditional theme. In set A, when a triangle faces up, there is an arrow pointing towards the triangle as well as a box containing a letter made up of straight lines only. When the triangle faces down, the arrow faces away from the triangle and the letter in the box is curved. In set B, when a triangle faces up there is an arrow pointing away from the triangle and the letter in the box is curved whilst when the triangle points down, the arrow points towards the triangle and the letter in the box is made up of straight lines.

Test Shape 1: Neither (to fit into set A the arrow should face towards the triangle)

Test Shape 2: Set B

Test Shape 3: Set A

Test Shape 4: Set A

Test Shape 5: Neither

Question Set 7

All the boxes look very similar, but the only pattern present is that in Set A, there is an odd number of shapes in each box whereas in Set B, there is an even number.

Test Shape 1: Set A

Test Shape 2: Set B

Test Shape 3: Set A

Test Shape 4: Set A

Test Shape 5: Set B

Question Set 8

This question is looking at the number of right angles. In Set A, there are 4 right angles in each box whereas in Set B, there are five in each box.

Test Shape 1: Neither

Test Shape 2: Set A

Test Shape 3: Neither

Test Shape 4: Set B

Test Shape 5: Set B

Question Set 9

Question 1 – Option A

This is an example of a type 3 question presenting you with a 'statement' between two shapes. If you consider the four squares together as collective, then the combined 'macro structure' rotates 90° anti-clockwise between the two shapes. If you apply the same rules, considering the four circles in the test shape as one large structure and rotate it 90° anti-clockwise, you will get Option A.

Question 2 – Option D

In the demonstration shapes of this type 3 question there are three objects – two squares and a circle. The object changes in such a way that the inside and outside shapes swap place (and size) so that the circle which was on the inside is now on the outside, and the black square that was on the outside is now on the inside. The middle square remains unchanged. If you apply the same changes to the test shape, the resulting new shape is Option D.

Question 3 – Option B

This is another example of a type 3 question. The demonstration shape is rotated 180° between the two boxes, which allows you to eliminate answer option C as the line within one of the boxes is orientated in the wrong direction. The next, and only other change, is that the two shaded boxes swap places. As such, the black box appears where the grey box was, and vice versa. If you apply the same rules to your test shape, only option B fits.

Question 4 – Option D

This is a type 2 question where you must find the next shape in the sequence. There are four items changing between each step: the triangle rotates 90° anti-clockwise between each step, the triangle changes colour from black to grey to white then back to black again, the star changes colour alternating between white and black and the star with attached circle rotates 90° clockwise each time (note the difference between the whole structure rotating 90° clockwise and the circle moving from one tip to the next). When you apply the earlier rules, the triangle should point up and be grey whilst the star should have the circle at the top (as it would have completed a full 360° rotation) and be coloured white. Only option D fits this description.

Question 5 – Option A

This is another type 2 question where the main change from one box to the next is colour. The small shapes change colour from black to grey to white then back to black again whilst the triangle simply alternates between black and white. There is no change in position or type of item. Following these rules, the next shape should contain a black triangle in the centre with the small shapes containing a grey square, black heart and white circle – option A.

Question Set 10

Question 10 is a type 1 question with a conditional pattern. In Set A, if the large shape has a horizontal line there are more unshaded than shaded small shapes, whereas if the large shape has a vertical line, there are more shaded than unshaded small shapes. The reverse is true in Set B where if there is a horizontal line, there are more shaded than unshaded small shapes whilst if the large shape has a vertical line, there are more unshaded than shaded small shapes.

Test Shape 1: Neither (as there is neither a vertical nor horizontal line)

Test Shape 2: Set B

Test Shape 3: Set B

Test Shape 4: Set A

Test Shape 5: Neither (as there are an equal number of shaded and unshaded small shapes)

Question Set 11

This is a type 4 question. In Set A, there is an odd number of total sides within each box whilst in Set B, there is an even number of total sides. There is no other pattern present, but as there are more shapes to evaluate for each question, the type 4 questions are more time consuming than type 1 questions despite being almost identical in most other respects. It is very important to make sure you read each question carefully to ensure you are looking for the correct test shape.

Question 1: Option A (1 side – odd)

Question 2: Option C (3 sides – odd)

Question 3: Option D (20 sides – even)

Question 4: Option C (11 sides – odd)

Question 5: Option D (6 sides – even)

CHAPTER 5

Situational Judgement Test

Overview

The Situational Judgement Test (SJT) was added to the UKCAT exam in 2013. It presents students with a range of hypothetical life, and work, related scenarios to assess how they deal with them. The scenarios focus on:

- Ethical and moral dilemmas
- Managing difficult emotional situations
- Conflict resolution
- Honesty and integrity
- Pressure and prioritisation
- Team working and leadership skills
- Communication skills

Situational judgement testing is becoming increasingly popular in the world of medicine. You will be regularly tested using SJTs throughout medical school, as part of your FY1 application, and in certain postgraduate speciality training programmes, such as General Practice and Emergency Medicine.

Format of the Section

This section consists of 69 questions split across 22 scenarios. Each scenario has between 2 and 6 associated questions. You have a generous 27 minutes (including 1 minute of reading time) to complete the section. This leaves you with approximately 23 seconds per question. Although this doesn't sound like much, students often feel that this section is the least time pressured in the UKCAT.

There are two types of task:

- Rating the *appropriateness* of a response to the scenario
- Rating how *important* it is to undertake an action in the context of a scenario

Scoring

The scoring used in the situational judgement section is completely different to the other four sections of the UKCAT. In other sections, the correct answer scores one mark. In the SJT, the best answer scores full marks – but subsequent answers may also score partial marks. You will therefore accumulate marks through the section, picking up more marks the more consistently you get the best – or close to the best – answer. Your raw score is then converted into a 'band', ranging from Band 1 (highest) to Band 4 (lowest). This is then presented as a standalone score. It is *not* combined with your score from the other four sections.

What does this mean? Each university will look at the SJT score independently from your scores for the other four sections. Many universities do not look at the SJT score. For those that do, a Band 1 or 2 score should be sufficient to meet their criteria. Some universities will instead use your SJT score as a 'virtual MMI station' that is combined with your interview score.

Top Tip: Always use your UKCAT score strategically. If your SJT score is lower than you hoped for, look at applying to universities who do not consider the SJT score.

General Strategy

In order to be successful in the SJT you must remember some golden rules that apply to both question types:

1. They are assessing your choice of actions, not the scenario. The scenarios are designed to be challenging and may involve you or someone else having acted irresponsibly. The aim of SJT is to assess how you respond to and deal with the situation. Someone could have done something awful in the scenario, but the way in which you choose to deal with it can still be excellent.

2. Never make assumptions. In SJT, it is tempting to keep asking 'what if…'. As a result, you might assume things which are not stated or implied. Do not assume anything to be the case, unless it is written down. Base your response purely on the facts you have.

3. You do not need any pre-existing medical knowledge. The UKCAT is meant to assess aptitude, rather than knowledge. The SJT is no exception. Although a basic understanding of how to deal with difficult situations and ethics will help you, you will not be expected to have any specific medical knowledge.

4. Always ask yourself: what does the examiner want me to do? Often, what we should do and what we actually do are completely different. Our judgement may become clouded,

as a scenario may be based around a friend rather than a stranger. However, it is important to stay impartial and consider the 'textbook' approach to tackling any scenario.

5. For each scenario you can use each answer option as many or as few times as you wish.

6. Each question within a scenario is completely independent from all other questions. Answers are not dependent on how you responded to previous questions and you should not take this into account when deciding what to do.

7. The actions provided are not 'complete'. Sometimes students are put off from selecting strong answers (such as 'very appropriate' or 'very inappropriate') as the action described on its own does not seem strong enough. However, you should never judge the response as if it is the only action taken.

A potentially useful resource to help you get into the right mindset of approaching Situational Judgement is the General Medical Council's (GMC) Good Medical Practice guide. You can access this on the GMC website: https://www.gmc-uk.org/guidance/good_medical_practice.asp.

Appropriateness Questions

Appropriateness questions ask you to rate how appropriate you think a response is, in the context of the scenario. You have four options to choose from:

- A very appropriate thing to do
- Appropriate, but not ideal
- Inappropriate, but not awful
- A very inappropriate thing to do

Strategy for Appropriateness Questions

Always read the scenario first. In the SJT, unlike other sections of the UKCAT, it is impossible to answer the questions without having first read the scenario. Fortunately, the scenarios tend to be quite short and don't take long to read.

Officially, UKCAT define the answer options as:

- *A very appropriate thing to do*: It will address at least one aspect of the situation.
- *Appropriate, but not ideal*: It could be done, but is not necessarily a very good thing to do.
- *Inappropriate, but not awful*: It should not really be done, but would not be terrible.
- *A very inappropriate thing to do*: It should definitely not be done and would make the situation worse.

Students often find it hard to choose between the various options. Getting to grips with how to differentiate between the answers can seem tricky. When you analyse the answers, you will frequently find that there will be combinations of positive and negative elements:

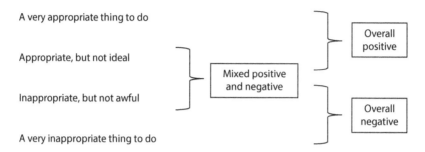

To help you decide on the correct answer it is best to adopt an algorithm. Firstly, you must decide if you think the action is positive or negative overall. The second step is to decide if the action is 'pure' or 'mixed', that is, are all components of the action positive or negative? Or is there a mixture of positive and negative elements?

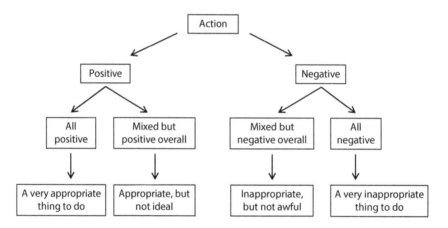

If you stick to this principle you will find it much easier to approach appropriateness questions. The real challenge arises when you have a mixture of positive and negative, and you need to decide which one is stronger.

Top Tip: Some students (and books) recommend always choosing the mixed options instead of the 'very' options, as even if you are wrong you are likely to be close to the correct answer and therefore pick up some points. This does not work!

Importance Questions

Importance questions ask you to rate how important you think a response is, in the context of the scenario. You have four options to choose from:

- Very important
- Important
- Of minor importance
- Not important at all

It is important that you understand the definitions of the terms correctly in order to be able to identify the correct response. Following are some modified definitions of the terms:

Very important: You *must* take this into account.

Important: You *should* take this into account.

Of minor importance: You *could* take this into account.

Not important at all: You should *not* take this into account.

Items that are crucial to undertake or consider are therefore 'very important'. Items which are important to consider, although not essential, are 'important'. If the item is something which you can take into account, but equally acceptable even if you do not, then it is 'of minor importance'. If the item is negative, and one that should not be enacted, or even taken into account, then it is 'not important at all'.

We will now look at some theory and questions designed to help you decide between the various answer options.

Choice of Vocabulary

It is vital that you pay close attention to the wording used to describe the action. This will help guide you as to whether or not the response is positive or negative. Look at the sample question in the following:

Example Scenario 1

You are a first-year medical student at a university, and to help fund your tuition fees you work part time at a local restaurant. You soon begin to notice that some items, including money from the tip jar, have started to disappear, and you suspect that one of your co-workers is stealing them.

How appropriate is the following response?

You decide to confront the person you think is responsible, threatening to report them to the management unless they return the items.

A. A very appropriate thing to do

B. Appropriate, but not ideal

C. Inappropriate, but not awful

D. A very inappropriate thing to do

Example Scenario 1: Answers and Explanations

In this case, the correct answer is 'Inappropriate, but not awful'. It is obvious that you have good intentions, both for yourself and fellow staff, to stop the stealing. You are also giving the person a chance to come clean and return the items. However, remember you only *suspect* they are responsible. As such, you could be offering an ultimatum (return the items or I report you) to someone who is innocent. There is clearly a mixture of positive and negative here.

Another major factor in helping you decide on the correct answer is the tone of your response. You 'confront' and 'threaten' the person in question. Confrontational and threatening behaviour is clearly not what the medical schools are looking for. It will be difficult to justify an overall positive response for actions that utilise these words.

You must therefore pay close attention to the choice of vocabulary used in your response. Following is a table of positive and negative words:

Positive		Negative	
Truthful	Propose	Threaten	Abuse
Honest	Encourage	Shout	Refuse
Open	Explore	Intimidate	Hide
Calm	Listen	Avoid	Blame
Support	Suggest	Confront	Shun
Recommend	Boost	Impatient	Accuse

If your action contains mainly positive words, then it is likely the action will be positive overall. Actions which contain negative words are unlikely to be positive overall. Changing the choice of wording has a drastic impact on the answer choice. Consider the aforementioned scenario again, but this time ask yourself how appropriate the following response is:

You sit down with the person in question, calmly voicing your concerns to him, and explore his side of the story.

All of a sudden, using words such as 'calmly' and 'exploring' gives a very positive tone to your response, making it very appropriate overall.

Refer to *Example Scenario 2* and answer all four questions in 1.5 minutes. Make a note of your answers before moving on to the explanations.

Example Scenario 2

Krish is sitting in his sixth form common room when a friend approaches him, visibly upset. He has been having trouble with his math teacher who he feels has been unfairly targeting him with criticism. He asks Krish for advice on what he should do.

How appropriate are each of the following responses by Krish in this situation?

1. Sit down and talk to his friend to find out more about the reasons why his teacher may be unhappy with him

    A. A very appropriate thing to do

    B. Appropriate, but not ideal

    C. Inappropriate, but not awful

    D. A very inappropriate thing to do

2. Tell his friend to go to his math tutor and ask him why he has an issue with him

    A. A very appropriate thing to do

    B. Appropriate, but not ideal

    C. Inappropriate, but not awful

    D. A very inappropriate thing to do

3. Tell his friend to ignore the issue and just continue to work as hard as possible in lessons

    A. A very appropriate thing to do

    B. Appropriate, but not ideal

    C. Inappropriate, but not awful

    D. A very inappropriate thing to do

4. Mention the problem to his form tutor and ask for her advice on how to proceed

    A. A very appropriate thing to do

    B. Appropriate, but not ideal

    C. Inappropriate, but not awful

    D. A very inappropriate thing to do

Example Scenario 2: Answers and Explanations

Question 1: A – A very appropriate thing to do

In this scenario it is important for Krish to know more about the situation, as it will help give him a better viewpoint from which to advise his friend. Additionally, discussing the issue may benefit his friend and help him realise why the problems are arising. This would be a good example of displaying both excellent communication skills and empathy.

Question 2: C – Inappropriate, but not awful

There are both positive and negative elements to this answer. On the positive side, he is encouraging his friend to tackle the problem directly and find out additional information. But on the negative side, this response would likely result in a discussion of a hostile nature and raise the level of conflict. After all, he's made the assumption that there is definitely a problem as the action includes definitive words: 'ask him why he *has* an issue with him' as opposed to 'ask *if* there was an issue'. But remember, there is a subjective element to the SJT, and that is why partial marks are awarded.

Question 3: C – Inappropriate, but not awful

While it would certainly be advisable to work as hard as possible, this response fails to deal with the issue at hand. The problem would go unresolved. Avoiding conflict would be a temporary solution that may lead to the issue resurfacing at a later date.

Question 4: B – Appropriate, but not ideal

This would be a very appropriate way of directly addressing the issue in a mature, non-confrontational manner. Form tutors are there to help with these types of issues, and throughout your medical career you will have supervisors there to help you when required. However, before speaking to his form tutor it would be wise to ensure his friend is happy with the plan of involving a staff member.

Communication Skills

Many scenarios in SJTs focus on communication skills, from dealing with angry or upset individuals to conflict resolution, and even breaking bad news. They are not just testing your intellectual ability but also your emotional maturity. In addition to verbal communication, it is important to consider the non-verbal communication aspects of a scenario. For instance, a scenario might tell you someone 'looks upset'. This is a form of non-verbal communication that needs to be considered, as it demonstrates a person's emotional state.

When deciding on answers, there are numerous factors to consider. Answers that express ideas clearly and sensitively are far more likely to be positive overall. It is equally important to consider the place in which the discussions take place. Consider the following scenario:

You are the passenger in a car being driven by your mother when her phone rings. You answer on her behalf only to find out that your grandfather has just passed away.

How appropriate is the following:

You immediately inform your mother so she can turn around and head straight to the hospital.

On the one hand, it seems that this may be an appropriate response as you should obviously inform her about what's happened. However, you must consider the time and place. Is it appropriate to break bad news while someone is driving? This is obviously a risk not just to you and your mother, but also all other road users. She will immediately become distracted and this may even lead to a crash.

The answer here is 'a very inappropriate thing to do'. Based on the decision to break bad news in inappropriate surroundings, you would be creating a risk to your mother and yourself, as well as other road users. It is vital that, in addition to communicating clearly and sensitively, you always consider the appropriate surroundings and best place to do so.

Some actions include seeking help or advice from others (example scenario 2, question 4). You will often be presented with scenarios outside your comfort zone, which you have not previously encountered. Seeking advice from someone more experienced is a very positive action, as it shows maturity and demonstrates that you know your limits.

> **Top Tip:** Although seeking advice is positive, be careful that the action doesn't involve you passing off your problems onto someone else. This would be a negative action as you fail to address the problem at hand.

In all communication-based questions, ensure you always within your remit. Common questions focus on scenarios such as the following:

'You are a medical student shadowing a GP when she gets called out of the room halfway through a consultation. The patient looks at you and asks you for their test results'.

It is crucial you always remember who you are in each scenario (the introduction will tell you). You need to base your responses on what you should be doing at that level. Clearly, in the scenario earlier, it would be very inappropriate for you as the medical student to release any test results to the patient.

Refer to *Example Scenario 3* and answer all four questions in 1.5 minutes. Make a note of your answers before moving on to the explanations.

Example Scenario 3

Sunny is a junior doctor, having just started his first placement, when he notices that one of the senior nurses has constantly been forgetting to put on a protective apron when going into potentially infectious patients' rooms. Sunny recalls how important this is from previous lectures, but also knows that this nurse is in charge of providing feedback on his performance to his consultant.

How important to take into account are the following considerations for Sunny when deciding how to respond to the situation?

1. That the senior nurse has been working for longer and has far more healthcare experience

   A.   Very important

   B.   Important

   C.   Of minor importance

   D.   Not important at all

2. The need to mention his observations to his consultant at their next academic meeting

   A.   Very important

   B.   Important

   C.   Of minor importance

   D.   Not important at all

3. The need to mention to the nurse his observation and emphasise how important it is to wear aprons

   A.   Very important

   B.   Important

   C.   Of minor importance

   D.   Not important at all

4. Continue to monitor it as he is hesitant to make a bad impression on a respected senior staff member

   A.   Very important

   B.   Important

   C.   Of minor importance

   D.   Not important at all

Example Scenario 3: Answers and Explanations

Question 1: D – Not important at all

In this instance, the fact that she has more experience than Sunny is neither the most important thing nor a mitigating factor. What is crucial is that, without his intervention, there is a risk to patient safety. So, while respecting the experience of senior colleagues is crucial, this is not something that needs to be taken into consideration. After all, even the most senior colleagues may need reminding of good practices!

Question 2: C – Of minor importance

While recognising a need to act, it may be more appropriate to involve a senior member of the nursing team instead, especially as there is a risk to patient safety. Furthermore, waiting for the academic meeting might take a while, and ideally this should be resolved sooner.

Question 3: A – Very important

This is crucial in this situation. It rectifies an issue that has the potential to endanger patient safety, while also treating a senior employee with respect. The ability to discuss important issues with colleagues in a mature and non-confrontational manner is essential in medicine.

Question 4: D – Not important at all

Again, the most important thing is patient safety. Failure to mention the issue or intervene is poor medical practice and is 'hiding' from the problem. This highlights how little importance this response carries.

Integrity, Professionalism and Probity

Integrity, professionalism and probity are key buzzwords used in medicine. As a doctor, you are expected to act as a professional, maintaining professional standards both in and out of work. These include:

- Acting with integrity
- Acting in ways that promote and maintain the public trust for the medical profession
- Taking responsibility
- Keeping up to date and providing the highest standards of care
- Admitting when you are wrong and reflecting on events

Many SJT scenarios are designed to push you on these issues. Answers which compromise your integrity and trustworthiness are always going to be negative. This includes:

- Not addressing the problems at hand in order to avoid conflict
- Actions which are illegal or violate basic confidentiality
- Any form of dishonest behaviour

Although it seems obvious that dishonest actions will be negative, SJTs can still create scenarios whereby this choice becomes difficult. Withholding information from someone is obviously negative. But what if it is done with their best interests at heart? Is it right to withhold certain details of someone's death in order to spare the feelings of their relatives? The simple answer, for the purposes of the SJT, is 'no'. Never withhold any information just because you want to spare someone's feelings. People have a right to know details, should they wish. Often, knowing what's happened will help with the grieving process.

Confidentiality

Confidentiality is a complicated area far above the level required for the UKCAT exam. There have, however, been questions which require a basic understanding of confidentiality in previous exams.

The purpose of confidentiality is that it allows patients and doctors to form a bond with trust. Patients feel free to disclose personal information, often essential for making the correct diagnosis, knowing that it will stay between them and the doctor. For the purposes of SJT you must respect this right. Any answers that involve distributing or sharing patient information to others is usually negative.

Although there are several instances when you may break confidentiality, for the purposes of UKCAT, the simple rule is that unless a person's life is at risk, you do not break confidentiality. If a patient has told you something which they do not want their doctor to know, then you should encourage them to allow you to tell their doctor by clearly explaining the importance. If you want to read more about confidentiality, a section on this can be found in the GMC's Good Medical Practice guide.

Refer to *Example Scenario 4* and answer all four questions in 1.5 minutes. Make a note of your answers before moving on to the explanations.

Example Scenario 4

> Roger is the captain of his sixth form football team. A teammate approaches him saying that the team's results have not been good of late and that he feels he should consider stepping down as captain. Roger has, however, been enjoying the role of captain and would like to continue.

How appropriate are each of the following responses by Roger in this situation?

1. Step down as captain immediately to avoid conflict

    A.   A very appropriate thing to do

    B.   Appropriate, but not ideal

    C.   Inappropriate, but not awful

    D.   A very inappropriate thing to do

2. Discuss with his teammate any issues he has with his captaincy and tell him he'll take them on board to improve

    A.   A very appropriate thing to do

    B.   Appropriate, but not ideal

    C.   Inappropriate, but not awful

    D.   A very inappropriate thing to do

3. Call a team meeting, tell the whole team his teammate's views, and ask for their opinion

   A.   A very appropriate thing to do

   B.   Appropriate, but not ideal

   C.   Inappropriate, but not awful

   D.   A very inappropriate thing to do

4. Immediately tell his teammate he will not be stepping down but that he appreciates his views and will work hard to address the issues he raised

   A.   A very appropriate thing to do

   B.   Appropriate, but not ideal

   C.   Inappropriate, but not awful

   D.   A very inappropriate thing to do

Example Scenario 4: Answers and Explanations

Question 1: D – A very inappropriate thing to do

As you go through your medical career you will constantly encounter challenges. Stepping down at the first sign of difficulty is not the ideal way to approach things. While stepping down may ultimately be correct for Roger, it would be advisable to discuss things further first in order to make an informed decision.

Question 2: A – A very appropriate thing to do

This is a non-confrontational and mature way to approach the situation. It takes into account the concerns of his teammate and gives time to come to a measured and well thought out decision.

Question 3: C – Inappropriate, but not awful

While it is often important to consult the opinions of others, it is very possible his teammate came to him in confidence and would rather his views be kept between them both. It would likely be wiser to consult the opinions of one or two senior teammates in a more private manner before addressing the whole team. Furthermore, this action may create a situation whereby people are forced to take sides, increasing the chances of conflict.

Question 4: B – Appropriate, but not ideal

In this scenario, Roger is within his rights to continue as captain. It also admirable that he wishes to rectify any issues his teammate has brought up. However, immediately refusing to even consider stepping down may be construed as very stubborn and uncooperative.

Teamwork and Leadership

Teamwork questions in SJT often focus on testing your understanding of the roles of team members and leaders, in combination with communication skills. Often, these communication skills will revolve around conflict resolution, where team members disagree with each other, or with a leader.

It is important to remember that all teams need structure and leadership. The role of the leader is to ensure the smooth running of the team, in order to achieve its task. To do this, the team leader must be prepared to listen to team members and involve the relevant parties when making decisions. This is a two-way line of communication. Listening is essential. Not only does it ensure decisions are discussed and more likely to be correct; it also makes the team members feel valued and appreciated, boosting the morale and productivity of the team.

In SJT scenarios where you are leading a team, it is therefore essential that you consider answers which involve you listening to, and taking feedback from, your team members. You will need to ensure workload is shared evenly across team members, and that people are undertaking the tasks to which they are best suited. There must always be a clear, two-way line of communication.

Refer to *Example Scenario 5* and answer all four questions in 1.5 minutes. Make a note of your answers before moving on to the explanations.

Example Scenario 5

Sarah is in her final year of medical school. As she nears a set of important exams, one of her friends, Nina, is beginning to become withdrawn and is showing signs of struggling with increased stress levels. This has been commented on by several of Nina's friends.

How important to take into account are the following considerations for Sarah when deciding how to respond to the situation?

1. The need to quickly tell a staff member about Nina in order to quickly deal with the problem

    A. Very important

    B. Important

    C. Of minor importance

    D. Not important at all

2. That she should discuss the situation with her other friends to see if they can come up with a solution together

    A. Very important

    B. Important

    C. Of minor importance

    D. Not important at all

3. The need to talk to Nina to find out if anything is bothering her

   A. Very important

   B. Important

   C. Of minor importance

   D. Not important at all

4. Keeping her distance from Nina to avoid exacerbating the situation

   A. Very important

   B. Important

   C. Of minor importance

   D. Not important at all

Example Scenario 5: Answers and Explanations

Question 1: D – Not important at all

It would not be advisable to bypass Nina by going straight to a member of staff. Nina could react negatively and become more likely to conceal any underlying issues she has, especially if she feels Sarah went behind her back.

Question 2: B – Important

It would be better to start by talking to Nina, finding out more information about what's going on. Usually, by widening the number of people involved it could complicate an already complex and delicate matter, but in this case the scenario tells you other people have already commented. Therefore, approaching it as a team is something to consider.

Question 3: A – Very important

By doing this Sarah is addressing the problem at hand and showing concern for Nina, whilst not threatening to get over-involved. As a result, Nina will be more likely to confide in her as she knows Sarah has her best interests at heart.

Question 4: D – Not important at all

This action, or lack thereof, may lead to problems snowballing, as Nina becomes even more withdrawn and feels that there is nobody she can talk to. It is important to demonstrate your emotional maturity and to be supportive, letting Nina know you are there to help her.

Pressure and Prioritisation

Pressure and prioritisation are intrinsically linked concepts. The more pressured you are, the more essential it becomes that you prioritise your tasks to ensure that the most important ones are completed. Pressure can be divided into 'acute' and 'chronic' pressure.

Acute pressure encompasses situations where there is a sudden event that puts people under pressure. This is often the result of unpredictable events and emergencies. SJT scenarios involving acute pressure often focus on work as a junior doctor, where you are suddenly faced with a large number of tasks, all of which seemingly need to be completed immediately. When choosing answers for scenarios involving acute pressure, look for those which approach the situation by:

1. Making a list of tasks to be completed

2. Prioritising tasks to ensure those which are important or urgent are addressed first

3. Regularly reviewing the list and reprioritising in case the situation has changed

4. Seeking help where required

If you're struggling, options which involve seeking help from colleagues or seniors are nearly always positive. Remember, seeking help is not the same as washing your hands of a problem!

Chronic pressure tends to be the result of numerous long-term tasks which all require significant time devotion. This may take the form of revision for exams, commitment to sports teams, and so on. To select suitable answer options for these questions, it is essential to look for options which break tasks into manageable steps (e.g. creating revision timetables and allocating realistic regular time devotion). They should set realistic goals and demonstrate perseverance, and ideally be balanced with stress relief, such as relaxation and sports.

Top Tip: If you are presented with a scenario where you are struggling, look for answer options which incorporate seeking help and advice from colleagues and seniors.

When deciding how to prioritise tasks, you can consider dividing them into those which are important/not important and urgent/not-urgent:

	Urgent	Non-Urgent
Important	Category I	Category II
Not Important	Category III	Category IV

Category I tasks are both urgent and important. This might be calling an ambulance if someone has collapsed, or leaving a burning building. These are tasks to which you must always allocate the highest priority (very appropriate/very important). They always trump other tasks.

Category II tasks includes those which are important but not urgent, that is those which require regular time devotion, such as revision or exercise. Category III tasks are the quick interruptions in life, such as answering a phone call. Category IV tasks include those which are neither important nor urgent, and which should always be given the lowest priority. These might include watching TV, playing computer games and so on.

Time for some practice! Try answering the following *21 Practice Scenarios* containing *68 questions*. There is a mixture of 'appropriateness' and 'importance' style questions. You have 27 minutes to answer all questions. Detailed explanations are provided. Good luck!

Questions

Question Scenario 1

Nigel is a work experience student on a ward round. He has just witnessed his consultant inform a patient that they have a form of lung cancer. Shortly after, he runs into the patient's daughter who was not present, she asks him how her mother is doing.

How appropriate are each of the following responses by Nigel in this situation?

1. Inform the patient's daughter he has not heard any news recently on her mother's progress

   A. A very appropriate thing to do

   B. Appropriate, but not ideal

   C. Inappropriate, but not awful

   D. A very inappropriate thing to do

2. Inform the patient's daughter that she has just been diagnosed with a form of lung cancer

   A. A very appropriate thing to do

   B. Appropriate, but not ideal

   C. Inappropriate, but not awful

   D. A very inappropriate thing to do

3. Tell the patient's daughter this is information he is unable to give and she should ask one of the doctors

   A. A very appropriate thing to do

   B. Appropriate, but not ideal

   C. Inappropriate, but not awful

   D. A very inappropriate thing to do

4. After explaining that this is information he is unable to give, offer to speak to the consultant and arrange for him to come and have a discussion with the patient's daughter

   A. A very appropriate thing to do

   B. Appropriate, but not ideal

   C. Inappropriate, but not awful

   D. A very inappropriate thing to do

Question Scenario 2

Peter is a junior doctor on a urology rotation. He finds that due to short inpatient stays he has a lot of free time on a daily basis with no jobs or patients to attend to.

How appropriate are each of the following responses by Peter in this situation?

1. Offer to help other junior doctors on busier wards

   A. A very appropriate thing to do

   B. Appropriate, but not ideal

   C. Inappropriate, but not awful

   D. A very inappropriate thing to do

2. Ask his consultant to schedule extra outpatient sessions for him

   A. A very appropriate thing to do

   B. Appropriate, but not ideal

   C. Inappropriate, but not awful

   D. A very inappropriate thing to do

3. Mention the free time to his educational supervisor and ask their advice

   A. A very appropriate thing to do

   B. Appropriate, but not ideal

   C. Inappropriate, but not awful

   D. A very inappropriate thing to do

Question Scenario 3

Nitish is one of two junior doctors on a cardiology rotation. When it comes to dividing jobs, Nitish finds that his other colleague, Ben, always goes for the quick and easy jobs, leaving Nitish with the harder jobs. Despite this, Nitish and Ben usually finish their jobs at the same time.

How important to take into account are the following considerations for Nitish when deciding how to respond to the situation?

1. That he should mention that Ben is being unfair to his supervisor

   A. Very important

   B. Important

   C. Of minor importance

   D. Not important at all

2. The need to discuss the pattern of behaviour he has noticed with Ben

   A. Very important

   B. Important

   C. Of minor importance

   D. Not important at all

3. That he should consider ignoring the situation to avoid starting a conflict

   A. Very important

   B. Important

C. Of minor importance

D. Not important at all

Question Scenario 4

Whilst buying a sandwich at his local supermarket, Vincent receives a £50 note in change when in reality he should only have received a £5 note. Vincent only notices this later at the bus stop, a five minute walk from the supermarket.

How important to take into account are the following considerations for Vincent when deciding how to respond to the situation?

1. To make a note of the error so he can return the excess change tomorrow when returning to the supermarket

  A. Very important

  B. Important

  C. Of minor importance

  D. Not important at all

2. The need to keep hold of the change without spending it

  A. Very important

  B. Important

  C. Of minor importance

  D. Not important at all

3. Recall what else he's doing that afternoon

  A. Very important

  B. Important

  C. Of minor importance

  D. Not important at all

Question Scenario 5

Alice is the junior doctor on the cardiology ward when a pharmacist approaches her saying that the dosage of a certain drug for a patient has been doubled by her consultant. The pharmacist says he has rarely seen this dosage used and asks Alice why, but she is not sure. Her consultant is not on the ward.

How appropriate are each of the following responses by Alice in this situation?

1. Change the dosage back to the previous dose

  A. A very appropriate thing to do

  B. Appropriate, but not ideal

  C. Inappropriate, but not awful

  D. A very inappropriate thing to do

2. Offer to phone the consultant and get back to the pharmacist as soon as possible

    A. A very appropriate thing to do

    B. Appropriate, but not ideal

    C. Inappropriate, but not awful

    D. A very inappropriate thing to do

3. As her consultant is very experienced and knowledgeable, decide to keep the dose unchanged

    A. A very appropriate thing to do

    B. Appropriate, but not ideal

    C. Inappropriate, but not awful

    D. A very inappropriate thing to do

Question Scenario 6

Sam is walking home one evening when he witnesses a car bumping into and scratching a parked car outside a house whilst trying to park, causing minor damage to both vehicles. The driver, who appears unhurt, drives away without leaving a note, but Sam is able to note his license plate number.

How important to take into account are the following considerations for Sam when deciding how to respond to the situation?

1. The need to immediately call 999 to report the car crash

    A. Very important

    B. Important

    C. Of minor importance

    D. Not important at all

2. Whether or not anyone was injured in the accident

    A. Very important

    B. Important

    C. Of minor importance

    D. Not important at all

3. The need to inform the owners of the parked car of the events and provide them with the license plate number

    A. Very important

    B. Important

    C. Of minor importance

    D. Not important at all

Question Scenario 7

Nancy is working a weekend job as a shop assistant and she spots a good friend, Pippa, attempting to steal a pair of jeans from the display. She knows that Pippa's family have had money troubles recently and she has never done anything like this before.

How appropriate are each of the following responses by Nancy in this situation?

1. As she sympathises with Pippa's situation, pretend not to see her

   A. A very appropriate thing to do

   B. Appropriate, but not ideal

   C. Inappropriate, but not awful

   D. A very inappropriate thing to do

2. Rush over to Pippa and tell her to put the jeans back and offer to speak to her after the shift

   A. A very appropriate thing to do

   B. Appropriate, but not idea

   C. Inappropriate, but not awful

   D. A very inappropriate thing to do

3. Alert the store supervisor to the attempted theft but explain Pippa is her friend and that this is out of character for her

   A. A very appropriate thing to do

   B. Appropriate, but not ideal

   C. Inappropriate, but not awful

   D. A very inappropriate thing to do

Question Scenario 8

Daniel is a medical student on a surgical ward. He has a very important football game for the medical school which he cannot be late for. The time for the football game is also specifically set in his timetable. The ward is swamped with work and as Daniel is about to leave, the consultant kindly asks if he wouldn't mind staying behind for a couple of hours to help.

How appropriate are each of the following responses by Daniel in this situation?

1. Agree to stay and help the consultant but missing the football match

   A. A very appropriate thing to do

   B. Appropriate, but not ideal

   C. Inappropriate, but not awful

   D. A very inappropriate thing to do

2. Inform the consultant he is unable to stay due to an important prior engagement

    A. A very appropriate thing to do

    B. Appropriate, but not ideal

    C. Inappropriate, but not awful

    D. A very inappropriate thing to do

3. Inform the consultant he is unable to stay but offer to help stay later tomorrow if required as he will be free that afternoon

    A. A very appropriate thing to do

    B. Appropriate, but not ideal

    C. Inappropriate, but not awful

    D. A very inappropriate thing to do

Question Scenario 9

Huw is preparing for an important two-person A-level presentation to be given later that day when his partner, Mike, calls him to say he will be unable to attend as he is unwell. However, on a social media site, photos of Mike at a party last night have been posted just moments ago.

How important to take into account are the following considerations for Huw when deciding how to respond to the situation?

1. The reasons for why Mike is unwell

    A. Very important

    B. Important

    C. Of minor importance

    D. Not important at all

2. Involving a fellow student for advice on how to proceed as Huw is unsure

    A. Very important

    B. Important

    C. Of minor importance

    D. Not important at all

3. The need for the teacher to know that Mike has rung in sick despite attending a party the previous day

    A. Very important

    B. Important

    C. Of minor importance

    D. Not important at all

Question Scenario 10

Phil has just been set a very tough but important essay in his AS-level economics class and is finding it very difficult to prepare for it. A friend, Moira, in the year above remarks that she did the same essay last year and did very well. Moira asks Phil if he would like to see her essay.

How appropriate are each of the following responses by Phil in this situation?

1. Thank Moira for the offer but instead ask if she could spend an hour teaching him some key points

   A. A very appropriate thing to do

   B. Appropriate, but not ideal

   C. Inappropriate, but not awful

   D. A very inappropriate thing to do

2. Accept the copy of the essay and memorise just a few of the key points to use in his essay

   A. A very appropriate thing to do

   B. Appropriate, but not ideal

   C. Inappropriate, but not awful

   D. A very inappropriate thing to do

3. Decline the offer and continue to prepare for the essay as he was before

   A. A very appropriate thing to do

   B. Appropriate, but not ideal

   C. Inappropriate, but not awful

   D. A very inappropriate thing to do

Question Scenario 11

Ellie is a first-year junior doctor sent to take blood from an elderly patient who previously had leukaemia. From the initial results in the notes she can see it is highly likely there has been a recurrence of his leukaemia, but not all of the tests have been completed. The patient asks Ellie if his leukaemia has come back.

How appropriate are each of the following responses by Ellie in this situation?

1. Explain to the patient that she doesn't have all his results but will speak to him once she does

   A. A very appropriate thing to do

   B. Appropriate, but not ideal

   C. Inappropriate, but not awful

   D. A very inappropriate thing to do

2. Inform the patient that the leukaemia has most likely returned but the tests are yet to be finished

   A. A very appropriate thing to do

   B. Appropriate, but not ideal

   C. Inappropriate, but not awful

   D. A very inappropriate thing to do

3. Inform the patient the leukaemia has not returned

   A. A very appropriate thing to do

   B. Appropriate, but not ideal

   C. Inappropriate, but not awful

   D. A very inappropriate thing to do

4. Explain to the patient that she doesn't have all the results yet but once she does she will ask a senior member of the team to come and speak with him

   A. A very appropriate thing to do

   B. Appropriate, but not ideal

   C. Inappropriate, but not awful

   D. A very inappropriate thing to do

Question Scenario 12

Mary is volunteering at her local elderly care home on a Saturday afternoon. What had started as a friendly discussion between two residents has become confrontational and threatens to turn physical.

How important is it to take into account the following considerations for Mary when deciding how to respond to the situation?

1. The need to talk to the residents and resolve the situation herself

   A. Very important

   B. Important

   C. Of minor importance

   D. Not important at all

2. Involving a nearby staff nurse to help diffuse the situation

   A. Very important

   B. Important

   C. Of minor importance

   D. Not important at all

3. After the incident is dealt with, encourage the two residents to spend more time with each other to work out their differences

   A. Very important

   B. Important

   C. Of minor importance

   D. Not important at all

Question Scenario 13

Pavel is on his way home after a busy day and gets off onto the tube platform. At the far end of the platform he sees a blind man struggling to navigate his way around and there appears to be no tube staff nearby.

How appropriate are each of the following responses by Pavel in this situation?

1. Wait to see if one of the fellow commuters helps him

   A. A very appropriate thing to do

   B. Appropriate, but not ideal

   C. Inappropriate, but not awful

   D. A very inappropriate thing to do

2. Go and find the nearest member of staff and alert them that there is a blind passenger who requires assistance

   A. A very appropriate thing to do

   B. Appropriate, but not ideal

   C. Inappropriate, but not awful

   D. A very inappropriate thing to do

3. Head over to assist the blind commuter as best he can

   A. A very appropriate thing to do

   B. Appropriate, but not ideal

   C. Inappropriate, but not awful

   D. A very inappropriate thing to do

4. As it has been a long day, head home in the hope that a staff member or commuter will go to help

   A. A very appropriate thing to do

   B. Appropriate, but not ideal

   C. Inappropriate, but not awful

   D. A very inappropriate thing to do

Question Scenario 14

A mother and her teenage son come to see Natalie, a junior doctor on a general practice rotation. The mother is very concerned and angry about an apparent change in his behaviour and can be heard arguing with him in the waiting room. She does most of the talking whilst the teenager appears subdued and uncomfortable talking in front of his mother.

How important to take into account are the following considerations for Natalie when deciding how to respond to the situation?

1. Try to get the son to talk more about his side of the story

    A. Very important

    B. Important

    C. Of minor importance

    D. Not important at all

2. Tell the mother to stay quiet as she is affecting her son's ability to speak

    A. Very important

    B. Important

    C. Of minor importance

    D. Not important at all

3. The need to try to separate the mother and son so they can talk separately in order to make them feel more comfortable

    A. Very important

    B. Important

    C. Of minor importance

    D. Not important at all

Question Scenario 15

Oscar is the junior doctor on a ward round when he realises that he has mixed up the first two patient's notes and has been documenting the findings in the incorrect notes. He is still mid-way through the busy ward round but knows he needs to correct the error.

How appropriate are each of the following responses by Oscar in this situation?

1. Informing his consultant of the error and letting him know he will correct it right away

    A. A very appropriate thing to do

    B. Appropriate, but not ideal

    C. Inappropriate, but not awful

    D. A very inappropriate thing to do

2. Waiting until after the ward round finishes and quickly correcting the notes

   A. A very appropriate thing to do

   B. Appropriate, but not ideal

   C. Inappropriate, but not awful

   D. A very inappropriate thing to do

3. Asking the other junior doctor on the ward round for advice on what to do

   A. A very appropriate thing to do

   B. Appropriate, but not ideal

   C. Inappropriate, but not awful

   D. A very inappropriate thing to do

Question Scenario 16

Henrik and Steve are both doctors. During a visit to Steve's apartment, Henrik sees he is taking medication obtained through falsified prescriptions. As well as this, Henrik suspects his habit is beginning to spiral out of control.

How important to take into account are the following considerations for Henrik when deciding how to respond to the situation?

1. Talking to Steve to find out why he is taking the medication

   A. Very important

   B. Important

   C. Of minor importance

   D. Not important at all

2. Reporting Steve to their consultant

   A. Very important

   B. Important

   C. Of minor importance

   D. Not important at all

3. The need to cover for Steve when he makes errors at work

   A. Very important

   B. Important

   C. Of minor importance

   D. Not important at all

4. Remaining supportive and encouraging Steve to seek help

   A. Very important

   B. Important

   C. Of minor importance

   D. Not important at all

Question Scenario 17

Fredrik is working as a FY2 doctor in an accident and emergency department. He sees a patient and diagnoses them with an illness which requires a complex treatment. He decides on a treatment, however, his FY1 colleague and a nurse disagree with the plan.

How important to take into account are the following considerations for Fredrik when deciding how to respond to the situation?

1. Trying to understand why they disagree with his choice

   A. Very important

   B. Important

   C. Of minor importance

   D. Not important at all

2. The fact that Fredrik is more senior than his colleagues

   A. Very important

   B. Important

   C. Of minor importance

   D. Not important at all

3. The need to quickly change his mind in light of the other opinions

   A. Very important

   B. Important

   C. Of minor importance

   D. Not important at all

4. Involving a senior doctor

   A. Very important

   B. Important

   C. Of minor importance

   D. Not important at all

Question Scenario 18

Tristan is the junior doctor on a ward round where he observes a consultant gaining consent for organ donation from the family of a seriously ill patient. The family, although seemingly reluctant, eventually decide to agree. Later on, Tristan bumps into the family. They tell him they felt pressured by the consultant and really would not like to agree to organ donation.

How appropriate are each of the following responses by Tristan in this situation?

1. Tell the family to take the issue up with the consultant directly as due to his level he is unable to help

   A. A very appropriate thing to do

   B. Appropriate, but not ideal

   C. Inappropriate, but not awful

   D. A very inappropriate thing to do

2. Tell the family he will let the consultant know about their concerns and ask him to speak to them again

   A. A very appropriate thing to do

   B. Appropriate, but not ideal

   C. Inappropriate, but not awful

   D. A very inappropriate thing to do

3. Explore the family's concerns and answer any questions that they have regarding organ donation as best he can

   A. A very appropriate thing to do

   B. Appropriate, but not ideal

   C. Inappropriate, but not awful

   D. A very inappropriate thing to do

4. Inform his registrar (senior doctor) of the problem as it is likely they are well equipped to deal with the situation

   A. A very appropriate thing to do

   B. Appropriate, but not ideal

   C. Inappropriate, but not awful

   D. A very inappropriate thing to do

Question Scenario 19

As one of the school prefects, Isabella is on patrol around the school. During the patrol she notices a younger boy is being picked on by some of his peers.

How important to take into account are the following considerations for Isabella when deciding how to respond to the situation?

1. Allowing the young boy to fight back against the bullies to develop independence

    A. Very important

    B. Important

    C. Of minor importance

    D. Not important at all

2. Antagonising the bullies so that they understand how it feels

    A. Very important

    B. Important

    C. Of minor importance

    D. Not important at all

3. Providing reassurance to the boy who was picked on

    A. Very important

    B. Important

    C. Of minor importance

    D. Not important at all

Question Scenario 20

Laura is running late for a train and is rushing to the station. On her way, she notices a wallet on the ground with a name and address tag on it. Stopping, even for a minute, will mean she misses her train and is late for the concert she is attending.

How appropriate are each of the following responses by Laura in this situation?

1. Pick up the wallet and take it with her, then return it to a police station after the concert

    A. A very appropriate thing to do

    B. Appropriate, but not ideal

    C. Inappropriate, but not awful

    D. A very inappropriate thing to do

2. As the concert tickets were very expensive and she does not want to miss it, rush by and ignore the wallet

    A. A very appropriate thing to do

    B. Appropriate, but not ideal

    C. Inappropriate, but not awful

    D. A very inappropriate thing to do

3. Stop to pick up the wallet and hand it to a good friend instructing them to hand it in to the police station

    A. A very appropriate thing to do

    B. Appropriate, but not ideal

    C. Inappropriate, but not awful

    D. A very inappropriate thing to do

Question Scenario 21

Afra, Justin and Archie are part of a fundraising team at school. They aim to raise £1,000 for charity through a series of events; however, Archie has consistently been missing events. Afra and Justin are concerned, as their team has fallen behind its target.

How appropriate are each of the following responses by Justin in this situation?

1. Demand that Archie leaves the team

    A. A very appropriate thing to do

    B. Appropriate, but not ideal

    C. Inappropriate, but not awful

    D. A very inappropriate thing to do

2. Ask one of his other friends to help with events in case Archie doesn't attend

    A. A very appropriate thing to do

    B. Appropriate, but not ideal

    C. Inappropriate, but not awful

    D. A very inappropriate thing to do

Answers

Scenario 1

Question 1: D – A very inappropriate thing to do

This is highly inappropriate as this response is essentially lying to the patient's family, which is never acceptable. Whilst it is a very sensitive situation, it is crucial to remain honest, whilst respecting confidentiality and not overstepping the responsibilities of your role. As such, the ideal response would be to state that as he is a work experience student and is unable to give any clinical information, but offer to find a doctor who can.

Question 2: D – A very inappropriate thing to do

This is also very inappropriate because as a work experience student, this is information he is not qualified to be giving. Furthermore it is highly likely he will not know enough about the patient or the condition to answer the follow up questions. It is crucial in medicine to know the limitations of your role and know when to contact a senior.

Question 3: B – Appropriate, but not ideal

Whilst this is honest and respects the limitations of the work experience role, it is somewhat insensitive and does not get the patient's daughter any closer to finding out what is happening with her mother. It fails to resolve the situation.

Question 4: A – A very appropriate thing to do

This is the 'text book' response as it does not involve anything outside of the remit of a work experience student's duties and is also proactive in trying to find a solution to this sensitive situation. It also involves good communication skills as the information is relayed in a sensible manner.

Scenario 2

Question 1: B – Appropriate, but not ideal

Although this response is very well meaning, Peter is attached to a specific rotation for a reason and thus should attempt to re-invest his time in a manner that will help his specific team. However, it is far from an unreasonable action.

Question 2: A – A very appropriate thing to do

This is an ideal response as it is pro-active and shows Peter's consultant that he is eager to help in any way possible. It will also help out his urology team in the outpatients clinic, making the schedule run more efficiently.

Question 3: A – A very appropriate thing to do

This is again a very appropriate response as educational supervisors are in a place to assist you with any issues relating to your training. It will also highlight an issue that can be addressed for future junior doctors on the same rotation, thus improving their future work environment.

Scenario 3

Question 1: C – Of minor importance

In a situation such as this, it is advisable to deal directly with the person involved and tackle the issue head on. Involving a third party is not important or necessary at this stage. If Nitish were to speak to Ben and he was still refusing to take into account the concerns, then this may be an important next step. However, if Nitish felt Ben to be intimidating or unapproachable, this may be considered.

Question 2: A – Very important

This is the most important step to take in this situation. The discussion should be in a mature and non-argumentative manner. It is important to get the viewpoint of Ben as it may be possible he is unaware of his behaviour. Also, the fact that they both finish their jobs at the same time means Ben partner may be struggling to complete even basic jobs and may need further help.

Question 3: D – Not important at all

Although, generally speaking, conflict should always be avoided where possible, in this instance it is far more important to discuss this issue that has arisen. As mentioned earlier, this should obviously be done in as mature and non-confrontational way as possible.

Scenario 4

Question 1: B – Important

Whilst the ideal response would be to turn back immediately, this action crucially has the correct intention of returning money to the rightful place after an honest oversight by both parties.

Question 2: D – Not important at all

This is not an important action and is very non-committal. It fails to show a strong intention to return the money; deciding not to spend the money in the interim is a poor compromise.

Question 3: A – Very important

Remember to read the question carefully. The ideal response would be to return to the shop with the change, however, in this case before deciding to do this it would be prudent for Vincent to first consider what else he has scheduled for that afternoon. This will allow him to prioritise his actions.

Scenario 5

Question 1: D – A very inappropriate thing to do

It would be risky and somewhat irresponsible behaviour to just assume an error has been made and change the dosage back to normal. In this scenario, attempts should be made to definitively find out why the dose was changed before making any changes.

Question 2: A – A very appropriate thing to do

This is the ideal response, as not only does it resolve the issue at hand but it is using her own initiative, and taking responsibility of the situation, which is always a great thing to do in all aspects of life.

Question 3: D – A very inappropriate thing to do

Just assuming that the dose is correct or incorrect is very dangerous and compromises patient safety. Even the most experienced clinicians are capable of making dosing errors so it would be wise to double check with the consultant as quickly as possible.

Scenario 6

Question 1: B – Important

In the event of witnessing a car crash it is important to contact the police, particularly if you have important information or were the only witness of the accident. As no one has been injured it would be more appropriate to contact 111 as 999 should be reserved for potentially life threatening emergencies.

Question 2: A – Very important

Whether or not anyone was injured is a very important consideration, as it allows you to prioritise your actions. As such, it must be considered. Had someone been injured, you would then need to call an ambulance and potentially try to administer first aid.

Question 3: A – Very important

This is very important to do as it is likely that without your intervention the owners of the car will be unaware of what has occurred. If you imagine yourself in such a situation, it is highly likely you would wish to know if it had been your car involved in such an incident.

Scenario 7

Question 1: D – A very inappropriate thing to do

Whilst it is natural to feel sorry for her friend, it is Nancy's duty to act in an appropriate manner and to ensure the theft does not occur as an employee of the shop. Ignoring a problem is never a good solution.

Question 2: B – Appropriate, but not ideal

This response addresses the issue directly and also offers to help out Pippa by speaking to her after the shift as well as helping her avoid the trouble she would have got herself in. However, as a member of the shop, it is important to follow shop protocol and not to act with double standards just because Pippa is a friend. The same principles apply in a medical career.

Question 3: A – A very appropriate thing to do

This response addresses the situation and involves correct escalation to the appropriate senior with provision of both accurate information and background information that the supervisor can choose to use, as they require.

Scenario 8

Question 1: C – Inappropriate, but not awful

Whilst it is admirable to want to stay behind and help it would be letting down all his team-mates if he were to miss the game. Furthermore, work–life balance is crucial and as long as he is fulfilling the duties of his role and not compromising patient safety, he is within his rights to attend the game. Although generally speaking it would always be ideal for medical students to help out in any way they can.

Question 2: A – A very appropriate thing to do

This, although failing to help with the situation on the ward, is a very appropriate thing to do in this situation, especially as the time slot for the football game is specifically designated in Daniel's timetable. He is being open and honest about his situation.

Question 3: A – A very appropriate thing to do

This is also a very appropriate response. Whilst still rightfully attending the football game, this response also shows initiative in offering to help at a later date, endearing himself to his consultant in the process.

Scenario 9

Question 1: A – Very important

It is crucial not to jump to conclusions as it is possible that Mike may have had a case of food poisoning from food at the party. Also, as he is Huw's partner for an important presentation, it is crucial that he maintains good communication skills and trust throughout.

Question 2: B – Important

If unsure, it is important to seek advice from an appropriate source. In this instance a peer is very much an appropriate person to ask. However, if Huw feels able to proceed alone, it is certainly not essential to consult the advice of a peer, particularly in situations such as this, where the best course of action is to discuss the issue directly with the person in question.

Question 3: D – Not important at all

It is crucial not to make assumptions or jump to conclusions. It is neither essential nor advisable to inform the teacher that Mike was at a party the night before, especially as it hasn't even been discussed with Mike yet, and there could be a legitimate reason for his absence.

Scenario 10

Question 1: A – A very appropriate thing to do

This is a constructive way to use a friend's help and does not run any risk of plagiarism. This would be a very appropriate suggestion.

Question 2: D – A very inappropriate thing to do

Whilst this may seem like it will help achieve a higher grade, this is dishonest and also blatant plagiarism. It shows a lack of integrity that is undesirable in those pursuing a career in medicine.

Question 3: B – Appropriate, but not ideal

Whilst this is undoubtedly an honest approach, it doesn't utilise the potentially great learning resource that has been offered by Moira. There is a difference between using materials and learning from them, and simply copying them. Throughout your medical career it will be important to seize all opportunities that help with your learning process.

Scenario 11

Question 1: C – Inappropriate, but not awful

Whilst this response is both honest and adequately non-committal, it is above a first-year junior doctor's responsibility to be breaking news such as this. It would be more suitable to contact a senior doctor.

Question 2: D – A very inappropriate thing to do

On occasion in a medical career, brutal honesty is not always the best approach. Sometimes situations need to be handled in an honest but sensitive manner. Breaking the news to the patient in such a blunt manner and before the completion of all tests is highly inappropriate. You also need to remember that breaking news about a cancer diagnosis is outside the remit of a junior doctor.

Question 3: D – A very inappropriate thing to do

This is extremely dishonest and one of the worst possible things a doctor could say in such a situation. It is always crucial to keep integrity and the patient's feelings in mind when dealing with such difficult situations.

Question 4: A – A very appropriate thing to do

This is the most appropriate course of action as it maintains honesty and does not mislead the patient whilst also offering to find the member of the team with the ideal experience to break the likely bad news to the patient.

Scenario 12

Question 1: C – Of minor importance

Whilst action needs to be taken to deal with the situation, Mary is still relatively inexperienced as a volunteer, and so it is more important to urgently inform the trained staff of what has just happened. Therefore, the need to resolve it herself is of minor importance.

Question 2: A – Very important

It is very important to get the attention of an experienced professional who has been trained in dealing with these situations. The nurse will also be familiar with the residents which increases the likelihood of successfully persuading the residents to keep calm. This is something which must be done.

Question 3: D – Not important at all

Although there are good intentions behind this act, it is possible that this could spark another argument between the residents, which is the last thing you would want to happen. Furthermore, this would be part of a longer-term solution and not necessarily required to resolve the current situation.

Scenario 13

Question 1: D – A very inappropriate thing to do

This is a very passive response and shows a lack of willingness to act and take responsibility for the situation. It is clear that the man is in need of help so it is important to act accordingly, even if those around are not.

Question 2: B – Appropriate, but not ideal

In this response, Pavel is somewhat active and uses his initiative to contact the member of staff. However, it appears the man is in immediate need of help and may require attention sooner, if possible.

Question 3: A – A very appropriate thing to do

This response brings immediate help to the gentleman in need and also involves taking ownership of the issue at hand. Likely, it would be a relatively simple task of helping the commuter navigate, and there is not necessarily a need to alert a member of staff.

Question 4: D – A very inappropriate thing to do

This is clearly an inappropriate response. It does not address the problem at hand, and assuming that the man will be helped is dangerous. In such situations we should take it upon ourselves to help directly.

Scenario 14

Question 1: A – Very important

It seems that only one side is being heard. It may prove advantageous to listen to the teenager to see if he feels comfortable talking and explore what has been going on.

Question 2: D – Not important at all

This could provoke the mother and further to limit her son's desire to talk to you. The action is also quite confrontational and demonstrates poor communication skills.

Question 3: A – Very important

It appears that Natalie is only hearing one side of the story and the teenager, for whatever reason, is not speaking up. It may be that he is reluctant to talk in front of his mother, so asking to speak to them alone may allow her to maintain trust, confidentiality and identify the underlying problem.

Scenario 15

Question 1: A – A very appropriate thing to do

This response involves taking accountability for the error, and demonstrating honesty by admitting culpability to the relevant person. It is also crucial that the notes are amended as quickly as possible because another doctor or nurse may read the erroneous notes and therefore do something that may endanger the patient with this mistaken information.

Question 2: C – Inappropriate, but not awful

This approach shows a lack of accountability and integrity and also endangers the patient's safety. Ward rounds can last for hours so it is imperative to correct the mistake as quickly as possible. But at least there is the intention to correct the entry.

Question 3: A – A very appropriate thing to do

Remember the answers need not be complete – just because Oscar asks for advice doesn't mean he won't also act quickly to resolve the situation. Seeking advice when unsure how to tackle a problem is an excellent skill desired in potential doctors.

Scenario 16

Question 1: A – Very important

There could be many reasons behind his actions. It is therefore very important to clarify why he is taking prescription medication before taking any further action, after all, they might be legitimately prescribed.

Question 2: D – Not important at all

Going straight to the senior member may complicate matters and drive Steve further into the use of medication. It would also weaken any bond Henrik had with him, and make him feel more isolated. Remember, he does not have all of the facts yet and making allegations can have profound effects on his career.

Question 3: D – Not important at all

This action could eventually lead to serious consequences if Steve continues to make errors and patient safety is seriously compromised. In addition, constantly covering for him will reduce Henrik's own work output and increase the chance he will make errors.

Question 4: A – Very important

By persuading him to tackle the problem straight away, Henrik could start Steve on the road to recovery. Knowing he is supporting him will help him realise his problems and improve his chances of success.

Scenario 17

Question 1: A – Very important

It is very important to discuss it with them because there may have been a key detail that he, or perhaps they, overlooked. An open dialogue and discussion, especially when there may be disagreement, is essential amongst healthcare professionals, and improves patient safety and outcomes.

Question 2: D – Not important at all

Whilst Fredrik may be one year senior to the FY1, he is not necessarily senior to the nurse, who may have many more years of experience. Equally, just because he is senior does not mean he is necessarily right.

Question 3: D – Not important at all

Just because he is outnumbered does not necessarily mean he is wrong. It is important that he defends himself because it could be that he knows something to be right but is struggling to convince someone else. If in doubt, he should first discuss the plan with a senior.

Question 4: A – Very important

When there is a conflict of opinions, it is very important to discuss the issues with someone more experienced, in this case, a senior doctor who can offer clinical advice. Seeking help is a positive trait.

Scenario 18

Question 1: D – A very inappropriate thing to do

This response fails to help the family and is also fairly insensitive as it involves refusing to help in a situation where he is able to do so. Also, it is likely that the family will be somewhat daunted by the prospect of speaking to the consultant given the earlier events. As such, he is not offering any solution.

Question 2: A – A very appropriate thing to do

This is a good response and involves the use of communication skills to help resolve the issue. It also gives an opportunity to inform the consultant of the situation, as he/she may not have been aware that the family was reluctant the first time round.

Question 3: B – Appropriate, but not ideal

It is possible that the reason the family is reluctant is that they misunderstood some of the details the consultant was trying to convey. By exploring their concerns and answering any questions, he is improving their understanding as well as gaining a better idea of why this issue has arisen. On the other hand, he is probably not best placed to answer these types of questions, so ideally this should be done by someone more senior.

Question 4: B – Appropriate, but not ideal

In this situation it is better to refer the issue back to the person who consented in the first place, not a new person. Also, as the most senior member of the team, it is likely that the consultant would be best equipped to deal with this scenario. However, informing the registrar is nevertheless an acceptable solution.

Scenario 19

Question 1: D – Not important at all

This won't achieve much. In fact, it will teach the boy to fight violence with violence. The boy should be encouraged to show he is a bigger person by not reacting to them. However, he should not be discouraged to protect himself if the bullies can't see reason and attack him.

Question 2: D – Not important at all

By antagonising the bullies, Isabella has in essence become a bully herself – solving violence with violence. Often, when bullies are hurt, they take it out on people in a lesser position than them, so this action should not be advised as it is likely to only worsen the problem.

Question 3: B – Important

The boy needs to have his confidence restored; this action may help him feel better about himself. However, you cannot be 100% that the bullies will not return and find other ways to retaliate, for example, by cyberbullying.

Scenario 20

Question 1: B – Appropriate, but not ideal

Whilst the end intention to hand the wallet to the police is good, it is also somewhat inappropriate to keep the wallet for a prolonged period of time without contacting anyone. Also, if there was a stop and search at the concert it is possible she could be found with what appears to be stolen goods. It is therefore advisable to act quicker in this situation, whilst balancing this speed with her own time constraints.

Question 2: D – A very inappropriate thing to do

This is very inappropriate as it avoids her responsibilities as a good citizen, as well as showing a lack of integrity. Whilst the concert may be important to her, she still has a duty to act in a situation such as this.

Question 3: C – Inappropriate, but not awful

Whilst this will likely ensure the wallet gets to the police station as quickly as possible, this response involves handing the responsibility off to someone else rather than taking accountability herself. Also, whilst she may be trusting a good friend, she cannot be entirely sure what he or she may do. Therefore, the response is still highly uncertain.

Scenario 21

Question 1: D – A very inappropriate thing to do

Demanding that Archie leaves the team is inappropriate. Firstly, 'demand' is a strong and confrontational word. Secondly, they do not know the reasons for why Archie has been missing events. It could be legitimate – perhaps he was unaware or perhaps there are personal issues the rest of the team is unaware of. By not first finding out the underlying reasons they are making assumptions.

Question 2: C – Inappropriate, but not awful

The scenario states that they are a team, so any decision, such as involving another person, should be a team decision. There is no indication that Afra, or Archie for that matter, is aware of this decision. It also doesn't tackle the underlying problem with Archie, but simply masks it. It is, however, at least an attempt at providing a temporary solution to the problem.

Index